Di
Ma

M000201193

Asthma

Fourth Edition

Mani S. Kavuru, MD

Professor and Division Chief
Pulmonary and Critical Care Medicine
Brody School of Medicine
East Carolina University

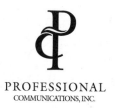

PROFESSIONAL
COMMUNICATIONS, INC.

Professional Communications, Inc.
A Medical Publishing Company

400 Center Bay Drive
West Islip, NY 11795
(t) 631/661-2852
(f) 631/661-2167

PO Box 10
Caddo, OK 74729-0010
(t) 580/367-9838
(f) 580/367-9989

For orders only, please call
1-800-337-9838

or visit our website at
www.pcibooks.com

ISBN: 978-1-932610-38-3

Printed in the United States of America

DISCLAIMER

The opinions expressed in this publication reflect those of the author. However, the author makes no warranty regarding the contents of the publication. The protocols described herein are general and may not apply to a specific patient. Any product mentioned in this publication should be taken in accordance with the prescribing information provided by the manufacturer.

This text is printed on recycled paper.

DEDICATION

To Joan, Vikram, and Priya.

ACKNOWLEDGMENT

I would like to thank teachers and mentors everywhere; I have been immensely blessed at all stages by interested and inspiring teachers.

TABLE OF CONTENTS

TABLES

FIGURES

1 Introduction

Asthma

Bronchial asthma affects 3% to 5% of the US population, making it a frequently encountered clinical problem in both the pediatric and the adult populations. It is a major cause of morbidity in the United States and around the world. Despite an increasing understanding of the pathogenesis of asthma, there has been an alarming increase in morbidity and mortality due to asthma during the past decade.

Although there is no general agreement concerning the reasons for this trend, the most important contributing factors may include:
- Delayed diagnosis
- Underassessment of the severity of the disease
- Undertreatment with anti-inflammatory agents
- Over-reliance on inhaled β-agonists.

Key developments in recent years in the field of asthma include:
- A firmer scientific basis for the concept of both inflammation and remodeling (further supporting current anti-inflammatory therapies)
- The "β-agonist controversy" continues to persist in different forms (see Chapter 4, *Pathogenesis: Role of Airway Inflammation and Airway Reactivity,* Pharmacogenetics section)
- New and evolving understanding of the notion of pharmacogenetics as being important for both assessing relative risk for subgroups as well as to identify responders to certain targeted therapies
- The approach of "combination therapy" has firmly taken hold in clinical practice

- Additional iterations in the delivery devices as well as increased use of dry powder formations has occurred
- A totally novel class of humanized monoclonal antibodies to IgE (ie, "biologic therapies") has come into use in selected patients with asthma.

In addition, the NAEPP issued updated guidelines in 2007. These guidelines have been incorporated into this edition.

The first iteration of the National Asthma Education and Prevention Program (NAEPP) guidelines were disseminated in 1991 as an Expert Panel Report (EPR-1). Over the ensuing 16 years, with a large body of accumulating clinical and scientific data, additional iterations were made (EPR-2 in 1997 and EPR-3 in September 2007). This substantial effort should be viewed as reinforcing the importance of this chronic illness, the ongoing challenges that clinicians (and patients) face daily, the modest progress that we have made, and highlight the continued need for advancements. Several key differences with the latest report warrant specific mention:

- As widely as the inflammatory basis has been embraced, the variability in the pattern of inflammation as well as the clinical phenotypes is emphasized.
- In addition to environmental allergens and atopic disease, the role of early viral infections, recurrent childhood wheezing, and family history predict disease persistence.
- The prior notion of assessment and monitoring has been further defined as disease severity (that affects the initial therapy), control (requiring monitoring), and responsiveness (therapies required to achieve goals). Both severity and control have been further defined in terms of impairment (current quality of life and overall

function) as well as risk (for future exacerbations of disease and permanent loss of lung function). Overall, these nuanced concepts emphasize that asthma may respond differently in different domains.

- Severity classification was revised to replace "mild intermittent" to "intermittent"; the concept that severe exacerbations can occur in any class of severity (including "intermittent") and that acute exacerbations can be mild, moderate, or severe in any category of persistent asthma.
- The peak flow monitoring is deemphasized for routine use but the emphasis remains on monitoring (either symptom-based or peak flow-based) as well as on asthma action plans.
- Although environmental control is recommended, there is insufficient evidence to recommend a specific strategy.
- Therapies continue to emphasize the primacy of anti-inflammatory agents.

Asthma should be viewed largely as an outpatient disease. It is likely that outcomes for chronic asthma will be improved by:

- Aggressive patient education in self-management skills
- Objective monitoring of early exacerbations
- Widespread use of anti-inflammatory therapy
- Use of new agents, ie, antileukotrienes.

Clearly, an aggressive program targeting high-risk patients is recommended. Recent trends in epidemiology, pathogenesis, and management principles will be reviewed in this text.

2
Definition and Classification

Asthma is a chronic, episodic disease of the airways with a spectrum of manifestations. In 1995, the National Heart, Lung, and Blood Institute (NHLBI) gave this working definition:

> *Asthma is a chronic inflammatory disorder of the airways in which many cells and cellular elements play a role, in particular, mast cells, eosinophils, T lymphocytes, macrophages, neutrophils, and epithelial cells. In susceptible individuals, this inflammation causes recurrent episodes of wheezing, breathlessness, chest tightness, and coughing, particularly at night or in the early morning. These episodes are usually associated with widespread but variable airflow obstruction that is often reversible either spontaneously or with treatment. The inflammation also causes an associated increase in the existing bronchial hyperresponsiveness to a variety of stimuli.*

Asthma is best viewed as a syndrome, and it is important to recognize the clinical features of the asthma syndrome (**Table 2.1**). All of these features need not be present for the diagnosis of asthma.

This inability to define asthma more precisely reflects the limitation of knowledge regarding the fundamental mechanisms operant in this disorder. Although there is some overlap in features between asthma and other chronic obstructive airflow disorders, such as chronic bronchitis and emphysema (**Figure 2.1**), it is crucial that one be able to distinguish between these problems (**Table 2.2**). For example:

**TABLE 2.1 — Defining Features
of the Asthma Syndrome**

- Episodic symptoms:
  - Cough
  - Wheeze
  - Dyspnea
- Airflow obstruction with a reversible component
- Bronchial hyperresponsiveness to a variety of specific and nonspecific stimuli
- Airway inflammation
- Tendency toward atopic and allergic disease

**FIGURE 2.1 — Chronic Airflow Limitation:
Overlapping Diseases**

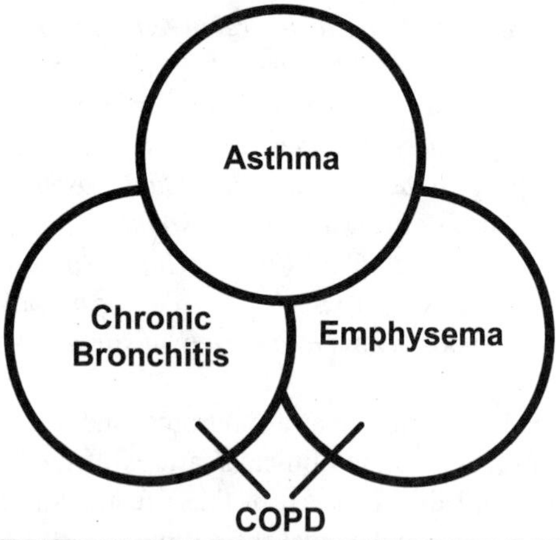

Abbreviation: COPD, chronic obstructive pulmonary disease.

TABLE 2.2 — Typical Features of Chronic Obstructive Pulmonary Disease

Feature	Asthma	Chronic Bronchitis	Emphysema
Age at onset (years)	Often <40	>40	>40
Smoking history	Variable	Heavy	Heavy
Pattern of symptoms	Episodic, chronic	Episodic, ? progressive	Progressive
Sputum	Mild	Severe	Mild
Associated atopy	Frequent	Occasional	Occasional
External triggers	Frequent	Occasional	Occasional
FEV_1, FEV_1-to-FVC ratio	Normal or low	Low	Low
Airway reactivity*	Almost always	Often	Often
Total lung capacity	Normal or mild increase	Normal or mild increase	Severe increase
DLCO	Normal or mild increase	Normal or mild increase	Severe decrease
Peak expiratory flow	Variable	Low	Low

Abbreviations: DLCO, carbon monoxide diffusing capacity of the lungs; FEV_1, forced expiratory volume in 1 second; FVC, forced vital capacity.

* Assessed by methacholine or histamine inhalational challenge in the pulmonary function lab.

Modified from: Kaliner M, Lemanske R. *JAMA*. 1992;268:2815.

- Asthma typically occurs in younger individuals.
- Exercise tolerance and spirometric parameters are much better preserved between episodes in asthmatics than in individuals with emphysema or chronic bronchitis.
- Asthma is sometimes classified as "extrinsic" or "intrinsic;" this distinction is of arguable clinical utility in the usual adult asthmatic (**Table 2.3**). The presence of extrinsic features may be helpful in solidifying an initial diagnosis of asthma.

Atopy, or the inherited ability to produce significant amounts of antigen-specific immunoglobulin E (IgE) antibody, is frequently present in younger asthmatics with extrinsic asthma. A clinical marker for atopy is a positive wheal-and-flare reaction to the intradermal administration of common allergens. Atopy and asthma are overlapping conditions, but each can occur without the other.

TABLE 2.3 — Comparison of Extrinsic and Intrinsic Asthma		
	Extrinsic	**Intrinsic**
Age at onset (years)	<18	>18
Seasonal variability	+++	+
Definable external triggers	+++	+
Atopic (ie, positive skin tests)	+++	+
Family history	++	+

SUGGESTED READING

American Thoracic Society statement: Standards for the diagnosis and care of patients with chronic obstructive pulmonary disease. *Am J Respir Crit Care Med.* 1995;152(suppl):S78-S121.

Asthma: the important questions–part 2. *Am Rev Respir Dis.* 1992;146:1349-1366.

Barnes PJ. A new approach to the treatment of asthma. *N Engl J Med.* 1989;321:1517-1527.

British Thoracic Society. Guidelines for management of asthma in adults. I–Chronic persistent asthma. *Br Med J.* 1990;301:651-653.

Clinical Practice Guidelines. Expert Panel Report 2: Guidelines for the Diagnosis and Management of Asthma. Bethesda, Md: US Dept of Health and Human Service, Public Health Service, National Institutes of Health, National Heart, Lung, and Blood Institute; 1997. NIH publication 97-4051.

Kaliner M, Lemanske R. Rhinitis and asthma. *JAMA.* 1992;268:2807-2829.

McFadden ER Jr, Gilbert IA. Asthma. *N Engl J Med.* 1992;327:1928-1937.

National Heart, Lung, and Blood Institute. National Institutes of Health. International consensus report on diagnosis and treatment of asthma. *Eur Respir J.* 1992;5:601-641. Publication 92-3091.

3

Epidemiology and Natural History

Recent Trends in the Epidemiology of Asthma

The most recent data from the National Center for Health Statistics indicate that in 2005, there were 22 million people who currently had asthma, including 15.7 million adults (7.2% of all adults) and 7.2 million children (8.9% of all children). Females were about 7% more likely than males to have ever been diagnosed with asthma, but among children from birth to 17 years of age, males were more likely to have an asthma diagnosis. Estimates of current asthma prevalence include people who have been diagnosed with asthma by a health professional and who still have asthma. Rates decreased with age. Females had a 30% higher prevalence compared with males. However, this pattern was reversed among children. The current asthma prevalence rate for boys from birth to 17 years of age is 30% higher than the rate among girls. Of these patients, 12 million people had experienced an asthma attack in the previous year. That is, about 60% of the people who had asthma at the time of the survey had an asthma attack in the previous year.

In 2004, there were 14.6 million outpatient asthma visits to private physician's offices and hospital outpatient departments and 1.8 million hospital emergency department visits. In 2005, there were 497,000 asthma hospitalizations. Hospitalizations were highest among children from birth to 4 years of age; the asthma hospitalization rate for blacks was 225% higher than for whites. Females had a hospitalization rate about 35% higher than males.

While the number of deaths due to asthma in the United States decreased to a low of 1674 in 1977, the annual age-adjusted death rate for asthma (as the underlying cause of death) increased 40% from 13.4 /1 million population (3154 deaths) in 1982 to 18.8/1 million (5106 deaths) in 1991. However, the death rate decreased again in 2002 to 4261 people, or 15/1 million. The death rate due to asthma decreased again in 2004 to 3780 (13/1 million). Non-Hispanic blacks were the most likely to die from asthma and had an asthma death rate >200% higher than non-Hispanic whites and 160% higher than Hispanics. The asthma death rate among females was about 40% higher than among males.

Risk Factors for Asthma-Related Deaths

There are numerous retrospective studies that have examined the circumstances of asthma-related deaths. Also, there are several case-control studies of patients who died because of asthma compared with matched survivors. The evolving consensus from these studies is that there are several risk factors that contribute to fatal asthma (**Table 3.1**):

- History of serious asthma requiring emergency department visits or mechanical ventilation
- Factors that may interfere with compliance and access to medical care
- Inadequate objective assessment of asthma severity by pulmonary function testing or peak-flow measurements
- Inadequate treatment with anti-inflammatory therapy and overreliance on inhaled β-agonists.

TABLE 3.1 — Risk Factors for Asthma Mortality

- History of prior serious asthma, including:
  - Emergency department visits
  - ICU stay
  - Mechanical ventilation
- Factors that may interfere with access to medical care and compliance, including:
  - Lower socioeconomic setting
  - Inner-city dwellers
  - Black, Hispanic groups
  - Substance abuse
- Inadequate objective assessment of asthma severity
- Overreliance on inhaled β-agonists
- Underutilization of anti-inflammatory medications
- Concomitant use of cocaine and bronchodilators

Abbreviation: ICU, intensive care unit.

Natural History

Our understanding of the natural history of asthma is limited. It is generally thought that asthma, unlike other chronic obstructive airflow disorders, does not inexorably progress from mild to severe disease. However, there are some studies which suggest that:

- Asthma alone can cause irreversible airflow obstruction
- The degree of obstruction is a function of the duration and severity of previous asthma
- Inflammation is present even in the mildest asthmatics
- Bulk of the "irreversible" loss of lung function may occur in the interval prior to start of anti-inflammatory therapy.

Data from an early study by Bronnimann and Burrows suggest that after the second decade, asthmatic subjects show a low rate of remission. The presence of severe respiratory symptoms reduces the likelihood that asthma will remit. Also, adults with a history of childhood asthma are at significant risk for future active asthma, especially if they have any persistent respiratory symptoms. In general, atopy is not useful in predicting remissions or relapses.

More recently, Porsbjerg and colleagues reported the results of a 12-year, prospective, follow-up study of the risk factors for the onset and remission of asthma in a random population sample ranging in age from 7 to 17 years at enrollment. In addition to an initial case history (including data on asthma, allergic diseases, and lifestyle patterns), airway responsiveness to histamine (AHR), lung function, and skin-prick test reactivity to a standard panel of 10 aeroallergens were measured. The point prevalence of asthma increased from 4.1% at the time of enrollment to 11.7% at follow-up. Asthma developed in 16.1% of subjects during the 12-year follow-up period, which was predicted by the following factors: wheezing in childhood (odds ratio [OR] 3.61); AHR (OR 4.94); allergic sensitization to house dust mites (OR 3.23); and dermatitis (OR 2.94). The presence of more than one of these factors was associated with a high probability of developing asthma during follow-up (61.5%). Conversely, asthma developed in only 4% of subjects without any of these factors at enrollment.

SUGGESTED READING

Bronnimann S, Burrows B. A prospective study of the natural history of asthma. Remission and relapse rates. *Chest*. 1986;90:480-484.

Gergen PJ, Mullally DI, Evans R III. National survey of prevalence of asthma among children in the United States, 1976 to 1980. *Pediatrics*. 1988;81:1-7.

Molfino NA, Nannini LJ, Martelli AN, et al. Respiratory arrest in near-fatal asthma. *N Engl J Med*. 1991;324:285-288.

Porsbjerg C, von Linstow ML, Ulrick CS, et al. Risk factors for onset of asthma: a 12-year prospective follow-up study. *Chest*. 2006;129:309-316.

Weiss KB, Wagener DK. Changing patterns of asthma mortality. Identifying target populations at high risk. *JAMA*. 1990;264:1683-1687.

3

4

Pathogenesis: Role of Airway Inflammation and Airway Reactivity

Early vs Late Asthma Response

Historically, asthma was viewed simply as a reversible, bronchospastic disorder with emphasis on smooth muscle contraction. While inflammation exists in mild-to-moderate asthma, it has long been known that patients who have died in status asthmaticus had extensive inflammatory changes of the airways, including:

- Mucus plugging
- Extensive epithelial sloughing
- Inflammatory cellular infiltrate of the mucosa and submucosa.

The central role of airway inflammation in the pathogenesis of asthma is being elucidated. Variable airflow obstruction and bronchial hyperreactivity (both specific and nonspecific) are central features in symptomatic asthma. The mechanism by which airway inflammation is related to bronchial reactivity remains unclear but is a source of intense research activity. Asthma represents a special type of inflammation of the airway that leads to contraction of airway smooth muscle, microvascular leakage, and bronchial hyper-responsiveness.

There are six well-described animal models of asthma and several human models of experimentally induced asthma that form the basis of current understanding of the pathogenesis of asthma. A classic model (Herxheimer reaction) is an allergic asthmatic challenge with an inhaled antigen to which the patient is sensitive (**Figure 4.1**). This challenge results in:

- A biphasic decline in respiratory function
- An early asthmatic response (EAR) occurring within minutes and resolving within 2 hours
- A late asthmatic response (LAR) that usually occurs within 6 to 8 hours and may last for 24 hours or longer.

The LAR, which appears to occur in 50% of adult asthmatics, is associated with increased airway reactivity to nonspecific stimuli (eg, methacholine or histamine) and inflammation in the airway lavage fluid. Pretreatment with β-agonists blocks only the EAR, whereas inhaled corticosteroids block only the LAR. Cromolyn sodium and nedocromil sodium block both

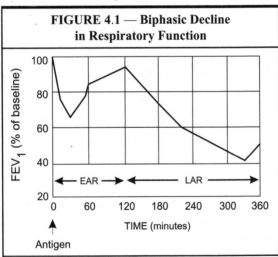

FIGURE 4.1 — Biphasic Decline in Respiratory Function

Abbreviations: EAR, early asthmatic response; LAR, late asthmatic response.

As measured by forced expiratory volume in 1 second (FEV_1) in an allergic asthmatic after inhalation of an allergen.

phases. In human studies, exposure to ozone and isocyanates results in LAR and influx of polymorphonuclear neutrophils (PMNs) in bronchoalveolar lavage (BAL) fluid. In the allergen and western red cedar (plicatic acid) model of asthma, there again appears an LAR, but the BAL fluid has an influx of both PMNs and eosinophils. These and other studies suggest that the specificity of stimulus and the species being studied affect the nature of the inflammatory process after exposure.

These observations in experimentally induced asthma have been extended to chronic stable asthma. Beasley and associates studied eight stable, atopic asthmatics and four controls. Endobronchial biopsies of the stable asthmatics showed extensive mucosal inflammation as characterized by:

- Epithelial sloughing
- Eosinophil infiltration of the submucosa
- Basement membrane thickening.

Also, BAL studies in these stable asthmatics showed the presence of a 5-fold increase in the shed epithelial cells and mast cells. Martin and colleagues evaluated BAL fluid in a group of asthmatics with nocturnal asthma and compared it with the fluid of asthmatics without nocturnal asthma. BAL was performed at 4 PM and 4 AM. A significant increase in BAL neutrophils, eosinophils, and lymphocytes was noted in patients with symptomatic nocturnal asthma at 4 AM compared with asthmatics without nocturnal symptoms. These studies suggest that airway inflammation plays a significant role in both experimentally induced asthma and in stable human chronic asthma. Numerous studies have suggested that the inflammation of asthma differs significantly from that of other airway or pulmonary parenchymal diseases by:

- The distinct absence of bronchiolitis
- Lack of fibrosis
- Absence of granulation tissue.

The reasons for this remain unclear.

Asthma Inflammatory Cascade

There is an emerging body of knowledge in asthma pathogenesis that implicates several different "players" in the asthma cascade (**Figure 4.2**). It appears there are inflammatory cellular, epithelial, neurogenic, and biochemical mediators that are important. It is likely that multiple cells and multiple mediators are involved in asthmatic responses in different individuals or even within a single asthmatic patient. A possible schema for the inflammatory cascade is that a stimulus (either specific or nonspecific) interacts with airway effector cells (such as mast cells or macrophages) to release a variety of preformed chemical mediators. These mediators (which may include histamine, prostaglandins, and leukotrienes) may produce the EAR by immediate effects on target airway tissue, resulting in:

- Airway smooth muscle constriction
- Hypersecretion of mucus
- Mucosal edema.

Simultaneously, lymphokines and other chemotactic compounds may elicit a migration of lymphocytes, neutrophils, and eosinophils to the site of degranulation and may activate the LAR, which may take hours to develop. These additional cells could subsequently produce mediators that may:

- Damage the respiratory epithelium
- Perpetuate or amplify the inflammatory process
- Stimulate afferent nerve endings and propagate a stimulus along other airways.

For example, eosinophils may release major basic protein, leukotriene C_4 (LTC_4), and platelet-activating

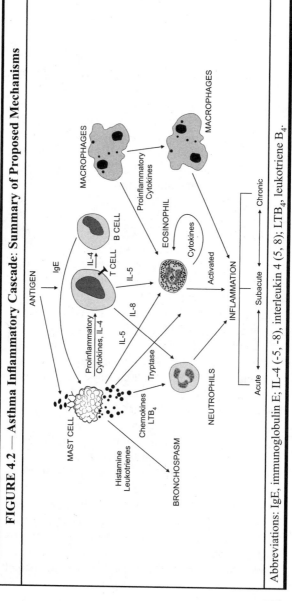

FIGURE 4.2 — Asthma Inflammatory Cascade: Summary of Proposed Mechanisms

Abbreviations: IgE, immunoglobulin E; IL-4 (-5, -8), interleukin 4 (5, 8); LTB$_4$, leukotriene B$_4$.

factor (PAF). Macrophages are a rich source of thromboxane (TXB_2), leukotriene B_4 (LTB_4), and PAF.

Numerous studies have recently advanced the notion that the T lymphocyte plays a pivotal role in the regulation and expression of local eosinophilia and IgE production in both asthma and allergic disease. Lavage fluid from patients with atopic asthma reveals expression of CD_4-positive lymphocytes (helper T cells). It appears that helper T cells can be further categorized as T_{H1} or T_{H2} cells based on the profile of cytokines these cells are capable of releasing. The T_{H1} cell produces interleukin 2 and 3 (IL-2 and IL-3), granulocyte-macrophage colony-stimulating factor (GM-CSF), and interferon gamma (INF-γ) which leads to delayed hypersensitivity-type response. In contrast, T_{H2} lymphocytes mediate allergic inflammation in atopic asthmatics by a cytokine profile that involves IL-4 (which directs B-lymphocytes to synthesize IgE), IL-5 (which is essential for the maturation of eosinophils), along with IL-3 and GM-CSF. Therefore, preliminary evidence suggests that atopic asthma is regulated by activation of the T_{H2}-like T-cell population.

Lipid mediators are products of arachidonic acid metabolism. They have been implicated in the airway inflammation of asthma and, therefore, have been the target of pharmacologic antagonism by a new class of agents – antileukotrienes. Prostaglandins are generated by the cyclooxygenation of arachidonic acid, and leukotrienes are generated by the lipoxygenation of arachidonic acid. The proinflammatory prostaglandins (PGD_2, PGF_2, TXB_2) cause bronchoconstriction, whereas other prostaglandins (PGE_2 and PGI_2 or prostacyclin) are considered protective and may elicit bronchodilation. Leukotrienes C_4, D_4, and E_4 comprise the compound slow-reacting substance of anaphylaxis (SRS-A), a potent stimulus of smooth muscle contraction and secretion of mucus. LTB_4 is a highly potent chemotactic factor for both neutrophils and eosinophils.

Several agents that interfere with leukotriene metabolism have recently been approved by the Food and Drug Administration for use in asthma (see Chapter 10, *Leukotriene Modifiers*).

Pharmacogenetics

Polymorphisms of the gene for the β_2-adrenergic receptor (AR) may be important in determining the clinical response to β-agonists. For the β_2-AR gene, single nucleotide polymorphisms (SNPs) have been defined at condons 16 and 27. The normal or "wild type" pattern is arginine-16-glycine and glutamine-27-glutamic acid but SNPs have been described with homozygous paring (eg, Gly16 Gly, Arg16 Arg, Glu27 Glu, and Gln27 Gln). Importantly, the frequency of these polymorphisms is the same in the normal population as in a population of asthmatics. Also, the presence of a gene variant itself does not appear to influence baseline lung function. However, in the presence of a polymorphism, the acute bronchodilator response to a β-agonist or protection from a bronchoconstrictor is affected.

Studies indicate that in patients with Arg16 Arg variant, the resulting β_2-AR is resistant to endogenous circulating catecholamines (eg, receptor density and integrity is preserved) with a subsequent ability to produce an acute bronchodilator response to an agonist. In patients with Gly16 Gly, the β_2-AR is downregulated by endogenous catecholamines, therefore, the acute bronchodilator response is reduced or blunted. In relation to prolonged β-agonist therapy (eg, >2 weeks), it appears that only patients who are homozygous for Arg16 who were receiving regularly scheduled β-agonist aerosol had a persistent decrease in lung function over time (eg, tachyphylaxis). These same individuals, when switched to as-needed albuterol, had no decrease in lung function, as is the case for

33

homozygous Gly16. Polymorphisms at the 27 loci are of unclear significance. Also, the impact of haplotypes (eg, variant genes linked at ≥ 2 loci) is presently unclear.

A recent study with transgenic mouse models using β_2-AR knockout as well as overexpression of β_2-AR has suggested an alternative molecular mechanism for the effects of chronic exposure to β-agonists and effects on airway bronchodilator response. Interestingly and unexpectedly, the mice with absent β_2-AR had markedly reduced bronchoconstrictive response to methacholine. The overexpressors of β_2-AR who had continuous β_2-AR signaling activity demonstrated an enhanced constrictive response. In addition, the overexpressors showed increased expression of a phospholipase C β_1-enzyme, which is thought to mediate the contractile response to methacholine. Overall, this study provides a new molecular mechanism to understand the effects of chronic β-agonist therapy on attenuated bronchodilator response (eg, tachyphylaxis).

To date, there are limited data on mutations involving the leukotriene cascade or corticosteroid metabolism. Polymorphisms of the 5-lipoxygenase (5-LO) promoter gene and the leukotriene C_4 (LTC_4) synthase gene have been described. Asthmatics with the "wild type" genotype at 5-LO have a greater response with 5-LO inhibitor therapy compared with asthmatics with a mutant gene. However, mutations of the 5-LO promoter occur only in about 5% of the asthmatic patients so it is unlikely to play an important role in most patients. An SNP in the LTC_4 synthase promoter gene (A-444C) is associated with increased leukotriene production and has a lower response to leukotriene-modifying agents. Fare less is known about genetic variability in the corticosteroid pathway. Polymorphisms in the glucocorticoid receptor gene have been identified, which appear to affect steroid binding and downstream pathways in various in vitro studies. However, polymorphisms in the glucocorticoid pathways have not been associated with the asthma phenotype or clinical steroid response.

SUGGESTED READING

Airway hyperreactivity. International symposium. October 26-28, 1988. Sendai, Japan. Proceedings. *Am Rev Respir Dis*. 1991;143 (suppl):S1-S84.

Barnes PJ. A new approach to the treatment of asthma. *N Engl J Med*. 1989;321:1517-1527.

Barnes PJ. New concepts in the pathogenesis of bronchial hyper-responsiveness and asthma. *J Allergy Clin Immunol*. 1989;83:1013-1026.

Beasley R, Roche WR, Roberts JA, Holgate ST. Cellular events in the bronchi in mild asthma and after bronchial provocation. *Am Rev Respir Dis*. 1989;139:806-817.

Bigby TD, Nadel JA. Asthma. In: Gallin JI, Goldstein IM, Snyderman R, eds. *Inflammation: Basic Principles and Clinical Correlates*. 2nd ed. New York, NY: Raven Press, Ltd; 1992:889-906.

Djukanovic R, Roche WR, Wilson JW, et al. Mucosal inflammation in asthma. *Am Rev Respir Dis*. 1990;142:434-457.

Kavuru MS, Dweik R, Thomassen MJ. Role of bronchoscopy in asthma research. *Clin Chest Med*. 1999;20:153-189.

Kay AB. "Helper" (CD_4+) T cells and eosinophils in allergy and asthma. *Am Rev Respir Dis*. 1992;145(suppl):S22-S26.

Larsen GL. The pulmonary late-phase response. *Hosp Pract*. 1987; 22:155-169.

Martin RJ, Cicutto LC, Smith HR, Ballard RD, Szefler SJ. Airways inflammation in nocturnal asthma. *Am Rev Respir Dis*. 1991;143:351-357.

Robinson DS, Hamid Q, Ying S, et al. Predominant T_{H2}-like bronchoalveolar T-lymphocyte population in atopic asthma. *N Engl J Med*. 1992;326:298-304.

Rochester CL, Rankin JA. Is asthma T-cell mediated? *Am Rev Respir Dis*. 1991;144:1005-1007.

Thomassen MJ, Buhrow LT, Connors MJ, Kaneko FT, Erzurum SC, Kavuru MS. Nitric oxide inhibits inflammatory cytokine production by human alveolar macrophages. *Am J Respir Cell Mol Biol*. 1997;17:279-283.

Wu J, Kobayashi M, Sousa EA, et al. Differential proteomic analysis of bronchoalveolar lavage fluid in asthmatics following segmental antigen challenge. *Mol Cell Proteomics*. 2005;4:1251-1264.

5

Clinical Evaluation and Assessment of Severity

Diagnosis

The history and physical examination of the patient are important to:

- Confirm a diagnosis of bronchial asthma (**Table 5.1**)
- Exclude asthma mimics (**Table 5.2**)
- Assess severity of airflow obstruction and the need for hospitalization (**Figures 5.1, 5.2**, and **5.3** and **Table 5.3**)
- Identify factors that might place a patient at particular risk for poor outcome, including death
- Identify comorbid diseases that may complicate the management of bronchial asthma (**Table 16.1**).

The cardinal symptoms of asthma include:

- Episodic dyspnea
- Chest tightness
- Wheezing
- Cough.

Some patients may present with atypical complaints such as:

- Symptoms on exercise alone (exercise-induced asthma)
- Isolated cough (cough-equivalent asthma).

It is essential to specifically inquire about nocturnal symptoms since this is often ignored. Key indicators for considering a diagnosis of asthma are shown in **Table 5.1**.

TABLE 5.1 — Key Indicators for Considering a Diagnosis of Asthma

Consider asthma and perform spirometry if any of the following indicators are present.* These indicators are not diagnostic by themselves, but the presence of multiple key indicators increases the probability of a diagnosis of asthma. Spirometry is needed to establish a diagnosis of asthma.

- Wheezing: high-pitched whistling sounds when breathing out, especially in children. (Absence of wheezing and a normal chest examination do not exclude asthma.)
- History of any of the following:
  - Cough, worse particularly at night
  - Recurrent wheezing
  - Recurrent difficulty in breathing
  - Recurrent chest tightness
- Reversible airflow limitation and diurnal variation as measured by using a peak flow meter, for example:
  - Peak expiratory flow (PEF) varies 20% or more from PEF measurement on arising in the morning (before taking an inhaled short-acting β_2-agonist) to PEF measurement in the early afternoon (after taking an inhaled short-acting β_2-agonist)
- Symptoms occur or worsen in the presence of:
  - Exercise
  - Viral infection
  - Animals with fur or feathers
  - House-dust mites (in mattresses, pillows, upholstered furniture, carpets)
  - Mold
  - Smoke (tobacco, wood)
  - Pollen
  - Changes in weather
  - Strong emotional expression (laughing or crying hard)
  - Airborne chemicals or dusts
  - Menses
- Symptoms occur or worsen at night, awakening the patient

* Eczema, hay fever, and a family history of asthma or atopic diseases are often associated with asthma, but they are not key indicators.

TABLE 5.2 — Asthma Mimics: Differential Diagnosis

- Other chronic obstructive airflow disorders:
  - Chronic bronchitis and emphysema
  - Cystic fibrosis
  - Bronchiectatic syndromes
- Anatomic, large airway obstruction:
  - Foreign bodies
  - Laryngospasm, edema
  - Vocal cord paralysis
  - Laryngotracheobronchomalacia
  - Benign/malignant endobronchial tumors
- Other conditions associated with wheezing:
  - Congestive heart failure (cardiac asthma)
  - Pulmonary embolism
  - Aspiration (gastroesophageal reflux)
  - Loeffler's syndrome
  - Factitious asthma (vocal cord dysfunction)

A detailed medical history of the new patient who is known or thought to have asthma should address the following items:

- Symptoms
- Pattern of symptoms
- Precipitating and/or aggravating factors
- Development of disease and treatment
- Family history
- Social history
- Profile of typical exacerbation
- Impact of asthma on patient and family
- Assessment of patient's and family's perceptions of disease.

In addition to the history and physical examination, an objective measurement of lung function by simple pulmonary function studies helps to confirm a diagnosis of asthma as well as to establish response to

FIGURE 5.1 — Classifying Asthma Severity and Initiating Treatment in Children 0 to 4 Years of Age

Assessing severity and initiating therapy in children who are not currently taking long-term control medication

Components of Severity		Classification of Asthma Severity (0-4 years of age)			
				Persistent	
		Intermittent	Mild	Moderate	Severe
Impairment	Symptoms	≤2 days/week	>2 days/week but not daily	Daily	Throughout the day
	Nighttime awakenings	0	1-2×/month	3-4×/month	>1×/week
	Short-acting β₂-agonist use for symptom control (not prevention of EIB)	≤2 days/week	>2 days/week but not daily	Daily	Several times per day
	Interference with normal activity	None	Minor limitation	Some limitation	Extremely limited

Risk	Exacerbations requiring oral systemic corticosteroids	0–1/year	≥2 exacerbations in 6 months requiring oral systemic corticosteroids, or ≥4 wheezing episodes/1 year lasting >1 day AND risk factors for persistent asthma
		Consider severity and interval since last exacerbation. Frequency and severity may fluctuate over time. 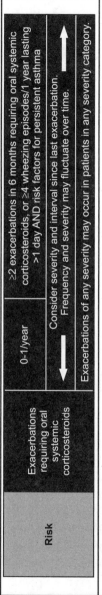	
	Exacerbations of any severity may occur in patients in any severity category.		

Abbreviation: EIB, exercise-induced bronchospasm.

- Level of severity is determined by both impairment and risk. Assess impairment domain by patient's/caregiver's recall of previous 2 to 4 weeks. Symptom assessment for longer periods should reflect a global assessment such as inquiring whether the patient's asthma is better or worse since the last visit. Assign severity to the most severe category in which any feature occurs.

- At present, there are inadequate data to correspond frequencies of exacerbations with different levels of asthma severity. For treatment purposes, patients who had ≥2 exacerbations requiring oral systemic corticosteroids in the past 6 months, or ≥4 wheezing episodes in the past year, and who have risk factors for persistent asthma may be considered the same as patients who have persistent asthma, even in the absence of impairment levels consistent with persistent asthma.

National Heart, Lung, and Blood Institute. National Asthma Education and Prevention Program. *Expert panel report 3: guidelines for the diagnosis and management of asthma;* August 28, 2007. *http://www.nhlbi.nih.gov/guidelines/asthma/asthgdln.pdf.* Accessed November 1, 2007.

5

FIGURE 5.2 — Classifying Asthma Severity in Children 5 to 11 Years of Age

Assessing severity and initiating therapy in children who are not currently taking long-term control medication

Components of Severity		Classification of Asthma Severity (5-11 years of age)			
		Intermittent	Persistent		
			Mild	Moderate	Severe
Impairment	Symptoms	≤2 days/week	>2 days/week but not daily	Daily	Throughout the day
	Nighttime awakenings	≤2×/month	3-4×/month	>1×/week but not nightly	Often 7×/week
	Short-acting β₂-agonist use for symptom control (not prevention of EIB)	≤2 days/week	>2 days/week but not daily	Daily	Several times per day
	Interference with normal activity	None	Minor limitation	Some limitation	Extremely limited
	Lung function	• Normal FEV₁ between exacerbations • FEV₁ >80% predicted • FEV₁/FVC >85%	• FEV₁ >80% predicted • FEV₁/FVC >80%	• FEV₁ 60% to 80% predicted • FEV₁/FVC 75% to 80%	• FEV₁ <60% predicted • FEV₁/FVC <75%

Risk	Exacerbations requiring oral systemic corticosteroids	0-1/year (see legend)	≥2/year (see legend)
		Consider severity and interval since last exacerbation. Frequency and severity may fluctuate over time for patients in any severity category.	
		Relative annual risk of exacerbations may be related to FEV_1.	

Abbreviations: EIB, exercise-induced brochospasm; FEV_1, forced expiratory volume in 1 second; FVC, forced vital capacity; ICU, intensive care unit.

- Level of severity is determined by both impairment and risk. Assess impairment domain by patient's/caregiver's recall of previous 2 to 4 weeks and spirometry. Assign severity to the most severe category in which any feature occurs.
- At present, there are inadequate data to correspond frequencies of exacerbations with different levels of asthma severity. In general, more frequent and intense exacerbations (eg, requiring urgent, unscheduled care, hospitalization, or ICU admission) indicate greater underlying disease severity. For treatment purposes, patients who had ≥2 exacerbations requiring oral systemic corticosteroids in the past year may be considered the same as patients who have persistent asthma, even in the absence of impairment levels consistent with persistent asthma.

National Heart, Lung, and Blood Institute. National Asthma Education and Prevention Program. *Expert panel report 3: guidelines for the diagnosis and management of asthma;* August 28, 2007. *http://www.nhlbi.nih.gov/guidelines/asthma/asthgdln.pdf.* Accessed November 1, 2007.

FIGURE 5.3 — Classifying Asthma Severity in Youths ≥12 Years of Age and Adults

Assessing severity and initiating therapy for patients who are not currently taking long-term control medications

Components of Severity		Classification of Asthma Severity (≥12 years of age)			
		Intermittent	Persistent		
			Mild	Moderate	Severe
Impairment Normal FEV$_1$/FVC: 8-19 yr 85% 20-39 yr 80% 40-59 yr 75% 60-80 yr 70%	Symptoms	≤2 days/week	>2 days/week but not daily	Daily	Throughout the day
	Nighttime awakenings	≤2×/month	3-4×/month	>1×/week but not nightly	Often 7×/week
	Short-acting β$_2$-agonist use for symptom control (not prevention of EIB)	≤2 days/week	>2 days/week but not daily, and not >1× on any day	Daily	Several times per day
	Interference with normal activity	None	Minor limitation	Some limitation	Extremely limited
	Lung function	• Normal FEV$_1$ between exacerbations • FEV$_1$ >80% predicted • FEV$_1$/FVC normal	• FEV$_1$ >80% predicted • FEV$_1$/FVC normal	• FEV$_1$ >60 but <80% predicted • FEV$_1$/FVC reduced 5%	• FEV$_1$ <60% predicted • FEV$_1$/FVC reduced >5%

	0-1/year (see legend)	≥2/year (see legend)
Risk	Exacerbations requiring oral systemic corticosteroids	
	Consider severity and interval since last exacerbation. Frequency and severity may fluctuate over time for patients in any severity category.	
	Relative annual risk of exacerbations may be related to FEV_1.	

Abbreviations: EIB, exercise-induced brochospasm; FEV_1, forced expiratory volume in 1 second; FVC, forced vital capacity; ICU, intensive care unit.

- Level of severity is determined by assessment of both impairment and risk. Assess impairment domain by patient's/caregiver's recall of previous 2 to 4 weeks and spirometry. Assign severity to the most severe category in which any feature occurs.
- At present, there are inadequate data to correspond frequencies of exacerbations with different levels of asthma severity. In general, more frequent and intense exacerbations (eg, requiring urgent, unscheduled care, hospitalization, or ICU admission) indicate greater underlying disease severity. For treatment purposes, patients who had ≥2 exacerbations requiring oral systemic corticosteroids in the past year may be considered the same as patients who have persistent asthma, even in the absence of impairment levels consistent with persistent asthma.

National Heart, Lung, and Blood Institute. National Asthma Education and Prevention Program. *Expert panel report 3: guidelines for the diagnosis and management of asthma*; August 28, 2007. *http://www.nhlbi.nih.gov/guidelines/asthma/asthgdln.pdf*. Accessed November 1, 2007.

TABLE 5.3 — Findings Suggestive of Status Asthmaticus in the Emergency Department

History
- Severe dyspnea, wheeze, cough
- Fragmented speech, sleep
- Difficulty walking 100 feet
- Increasing inhaler usage at home

Physical Findings
- Respiratory rate >30 breaths/min
- Heart rate >120 beats/min
- Accessory muscle use
- Pulsus paradoxus
- Silent chest
- Mental status changes

Expiratory Airflow Limitation
- Initial PEF <100 L/min (<20% predicted)
- Initial FEV_1 <0.8 to 1.0 L (<25% predicted)
- FEV_1 <1.6 to 2.1 L (<60% predicted) after therapy
- PEF <300 L/min (<60% predicted) after therapy

Gas Exchange
- Oxygen saturation <90%
- PCO_2 >40 mm Hg

Abbreviations: FEV_1, forced expiratory volume in 1 second; PCO_2, partial pressure of carbon dioxide; PEF, peak expiratory flow.

therapy. The most common and important indices of expiratory flow are:

- Forced expiratory volume in 1 second (FEV_1): the maximum volume of air expired in 1 second from full inspiration (total lung capacity [TLC]) to complete exhalation (residual volume [RV]); and
- Peak expiratory flow (PEF): the maximum flow that can be generated during a forced expiratory maneuver.

The forced vital capacity (FVC) maneuver (simple spirogram) may be graphically displayed either as a volume-time curve or as a flow-volume loop. An example of the normal spirogram is shown in **Figure 5**.4.

Spirometry in an asthmatic typically shows obstructive airway disease with reduced expiratory flows and volumes, which improve with bronchodilator therapy. A reduction in the FEV_1-to-FVC ratio is characteristic of obstructive airflow disease, and this ratio helps to distinguish obstructive airflow disease from restrictive disorders. Based on the recent American Thoracic Society criteria, airflow obstruction is considered reversible if the FEV_1 increases by at least 12% and 200 cc after two puffs of a β-agonist. Previous criteria required a 15% increase in the FEV_1 and did not require any given degree of absolute increase.

The shape of the flow-volume loop may provide insight into the nature and location of airway obstruction. **Figure 5**.5 and **Figure 5**.6 depict several characteristic patterns of the loop that help to localize the site of obstruction and distinguish asthma from asthma mimics such as upper airway obstruction (UAO). Normally, there is a limitation of airflow at high lung volumes that produces a sharp PEF in the expiratory limb of the flow-volume loop during periods of maximal flow. Both asthma and emphysema are examples of typical obstructive airflow disorders characterized by a concavity of the expiratory limb of the flow-volume loop with a fairly well-preserved inspiratory limb. The concavity is due to reduction in expiratory flow rates at low lung volumes. With disorders that cause UAO, either extrathoracic (ie, stridor due to vocal cord paralysis or edema) or intrathoracic (obstructing lesion involving the distal trachea), there is classically a plateau in either limb of the flow-volume loop during periods of maximal flow. With UAO, the shape of the loop is related to the level of the obstruction (above or below the thoracic inlet) and the net effect of pressures acting on the extrathoracic or intrathoracic airway, including the atmospheric

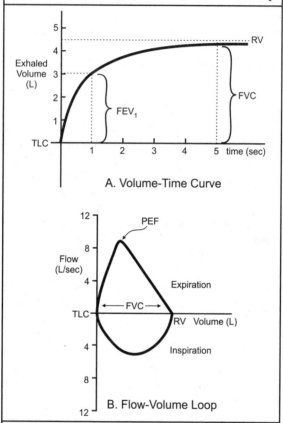

FIGURE 5.4 — Normal Spirogram Depicting the Volume-Time Curve and the Flow-Volume Loop

A. Volume-Time Curve

B. Flow-Volume Loop

Abbreviations: FEV_1, forced expiratory volume in 1 second; FVC, forced vital capacity; PEF, peak expiratory flow; RV, residual volume; TLC, total lung capacity.

pressure, intraluminal pressure and intrapleural pressure. The extrathoracic airway tends to collapse with inspiration (tracheal pressure is less than atmospheric pressure); the intrathoracic airway tends to collapse with expiration (tracheal pressure is less than pleural

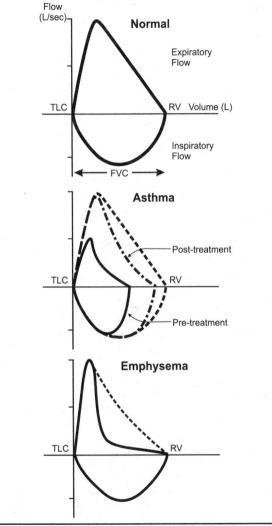

FIGURE 5.5 — Representative Flow-Volume Loops: Normal, Asthma, and Emphysema

Abbreviations: FVC, forced vital capacity; RV, residual volume; TLC, total lung capacity.

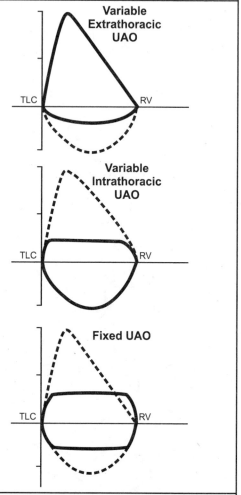

FIGURE 5.6 — Flow-Volume Loops: Three Types of Upper Airway Obstruction

Variable Extrathoracic UAO

TLC   RV

Variable Intrathoracic UAO

TLC   RV

Fixed UAO

TLC   RV

Abbreviations: RV, residual volume; TLC, total lung capacity; UAO, upper airway obstruction.

pressure). The flow-volume loop shows flattening of the inspiratory limb with variable extrathoracic UAO, likely due to a lesion involving the glottic or subglottic area. In contrast, flattening of the flow-volume loop limited to the expiratory limb occurs with variable intrathoracic UAO, usually on the basis of an obstructing lesion of the mid or distal trachea. "Boxlike" flattening of both the inspiratory and expiratory limbs of the flow-volume loop occurs with a fixed UAO due to any etiology.

When a patient presents with episodic and atypical chest symptoms, and the physical examination and simple spirometry are normal, a diagnosis of asthma may nevertheless be considered. These atypical chest symptoms may include:

- An isolated cough (cough-equivalent asthma)
- Mild exercise-related cough (exercise-induced bronchospasm)
- Dyspnea of unclear etiology.

Certainly, a normal lung examination and a normal spirometry would not exclude airway hyperreactivity or asthma as a cause for these symptoms. In order to define whether nonspecific airway hyperreactivity is a mechanism for such chest symptoms of unclear etiology, inhalational challenge tests are often utilized in the pulmonary function laboratory. A variety of agents may be utilized, but methacholine and histamine are the agents most often used. **Figure 5**.7 illustrates a sample response to methacholine or histamine inhalational challenge in a normal individual and in a patient with asthma. When the baseline spirogram is relatively normal, inhalational challenge may be performed by aerosolizing progressive concentrations of an agent such as methacholine or histamine by a dosimeter. This is typically performed as a five-stage procedure with five different concentrations. After each stage, the patient performs a spirogram. When there is a 20%

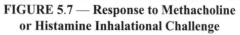

FIGURE 5.7 — Response to Methacholine or Histamine Inhalational Challenge

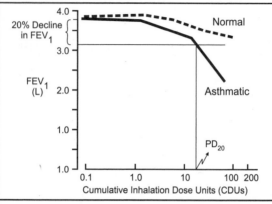

Abbreviations: FEV_1, forced expiratory volume in 1 second; PD_{20}, provocative dose of challenge agent required to produce a 20% reduction in FEV_1.

reduction in the FEV_1, the test is terminated and is considered positive for airway hyperreactivity. The provocative dose level of the inhalational agent required to produce a 20% reduction in the FEV_1 is labeled as PD_{20}. If the drop in FEV_1 is <20% after five stages of this procedure, the challenge test is considered negative for the presence of airway hyperreactivity.

Bronchial hyperreactivity as assessed by this inhalational challenge procedure is very sensitive for the presence of active or current asthma. A positive test is strongly suggestive of bronchial asthma. However, this test may be falsely made positive by a variety of conditions including:

- Chronic obstructive pulmonary disease other than asthma
- A variety of parenchymal respiratory disorders
- Congestive heart failure
- Allergic rhinitis
- Recent upper respiratory tract infection.

For practical purposes, a negative inhalational challenge with methacholine or histamine excludes active, symptomatic asthma as a cause for the patient's chest symptoms.

Factitious Asthma (Vocal Cord Dysfunction)

Over the past decade, several reports have described patients with functional vocal cord disorders that mimic attacks of bronchial asthma. The typical history involves episodes of wheezing and dyspnea that are refractory to standard therapy for asthma. These individuals may have wheezing that is often loudest over the neck, but the wheezing is often transmitted over both lung fields and may be misdiagnosed as bronchial asthma. During episodes of wheezing, the maximal expiratory and inspiratory flow-volume loop is consistent with variable extrathoracic UAO or fixed UAO as seen in **Figure 5.6**. The pathophysiology of factitious asthma, as noted by laryngoscopy, appears to be adduction of the true and false vocal cords throughout the respiratory cycle, including the inspiratory phase. During asymptomatic periods, both the flow-volume loop and the laryngoscopic examination are normal. Interestingly, methacholine or histamine provocation testing is usually negative for airway hyperreactivity. Christopher and associates described a variety of personality styles and psychiatric diagnoses in these individuals and suggested that factitious asthma is a form of conversion reaction. They described a dramatic response to speech therapy and psychotherapy in these patients with factitious vocal cord dysfunction. In general, factitious asthma should be included in the differential diagnosis of difficult-to-control asthma.

More recently, McFadden and colleagues described vocal cord dysfunction in elite athletes that presents as "choking" during exercise. This entity may be distinguished from typical exercise-induced asthma by several features (symptoms are maximal during exercise, absence of nocturnal symptoms are absent, and flow-volume loop is abnormal).

Evaluation of Severity

Numerous parameters from the physical examination and airflow measurement, either separately or as a composite score, have been evaluated to assess the severity of acute asthma (**Figures 5.1**, **5.2**, and **5.3**) and the need for hospitalization (**Table 5.3**).

An early study by McFadden and colleagues (1973) studied the relationship between clinical and physiologic manifestations of acute bronchial asthma serially during initial therapy in the emergency department (ED). Regardless of the initial presentation of the patients, when they became asymptomatic, the overall mechanical function of the lungs as assessed by FEV_1 was still as low as 40% to 50% of predicted normal values. When they were without signs of asthma on examination, FEV_1 was only 60% to 70% of predicted values.

This study reinforces the need for objective measurement of airflow obstruction during acute asthma. It is true that physical findings such as the following are generally associated with more severe airflow obstruction:

- Pulsus paradoxus (inspiratory decline in systolic blood pressure >12 mm Hg)
- Accessory muscle use, including sternocleidomastoid muscle retraction
- Respiratory rate >30 breaths/min
- Heart rate >120 beats/min.

However, none of these signs either alone or in combination are specific or sensitive.

Identifying High-Risk Patients and Hospital Admission Criteria

The most objective indicator of asthma severity is the measurement of airflow obstruction by spirometry, either by FEV_1 or PEF. Both the FEV_1 and PEF yield comparable results. **Figures 5.8** and **5.9** depict a sample PEF nomogram. A severe asthma exacerbation may be accurately indicated by:

- An FEV_1 <0.8 L to 1.0 L (<25% predicted in ages 25 to 65 years), or
- A PEF <100 L/min (<20% predicted in ages 25 to 65 years).

An increase in FEV_1 to >1.6 L to 2.1 L (>60% predicted) or a PEF improvement to >300 L/min (>60% predicted) after therapy usually negates the need for hospitalization.

Fischl and associates described an index that predicted relapse and the need for hospitalization in 205 patients with acute bronchial asthma. Of the 205 patients, 120 were successfully treated and discharged from the ED, 45 were hospitalized, and 40 were treated and discharged from the ED but had relapses within 10 days. A predictive index using a combination of seven presenting factors was developed:

- Pulse >120 beats/min
- Respiratory rate >30 breaths/min
- Pulsus paradoxus >18 mm Hg
- PEF <120 L/min
- Moderate-to-severe dyspnea
- Accessory muscle use
- Wheezing.

Presence of four or more of the seven factors upon presentation to the ED (prior to therapy) was 95% accurate in predicting the risk of relapse and 96%

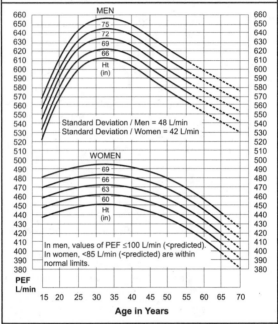

FIGURE 5.8 — Predicted Nomogram for Peak Expiratory Flow by Age

Abbreviation: PEF, peak expiratory flow.

Expert Panel Report of the National Asthma Education and Prevention Program. *Guidelines for the Diagnosis and Management of Asthma.* Bethesda, Md: National Institutes of Health; 1991:23.

accurate in predicting the need for hospitalization. However, subsequent prospective studies using this index failed to confirm these findings. None of these signs or symptoms, either alone or in combination, is specific or sensitive.

Chest x-ray adds little to the acute evaluation of an asthmatic. Hyperinflation is the most common finding on a chest x-ray, and it has no diagnostic or therapeutic

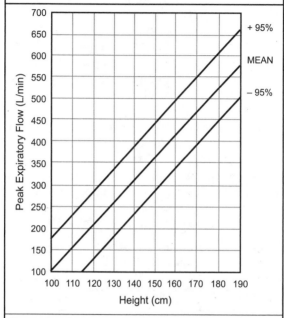

FIGURE 5.9 — Predicted Normal Range for Peak Expiratory Flow by Height for Men and Women

Expert Panel Report of the National Asthma Education and Prevention Program. *Guidelines for the Diagnosis and Management of Asthma.* Bethesda, Md: National Institutes of Health; 1991:23.

value. It should not be obtained unless complications are suspected such as:

- Pneumonia
- Pneumothorax
- An endobronchial lesion.

Nowak and associates prospectively compared arterial blood gas and pulmonary function measurements in 102 episodes of acute bronchial asthma initially seen in the ED. The partial pressure of arterial oxygen (PaO_2), partial pressure of carbon dioxide in arterial gas ($PaCO_2$), or pH did not separate those patients requiring admission from those that could be discharged. All patients with $PaCO_2$ >42 and/or severe hypoxemia (PaO_2 <60) had a PEF <200 L/min or an FEV_1 <1.0 L. In an elegant study by McFadden and Lyons (1968), it was demonstrated that alveolar ventilation remains relatively fixed until the FEV_1 drops to 25% of predicted, and at this point tidal volume falls, causing both minute and alveolar ventilation to drop. Initially, the $PaCO_2$ begins to return to normal, and when the FEV_1 is 15% of predicted, $PaCO_2$ retention begins to occur. In summary, arterial blood gases should be obtained only when indices of airflow suggest that severe obstruction is present. In the setting of acute asthma, when arterial blood gases are obtained, presence of normocapnia or hypercapnia represents severe disease that usually requires intensive care (**Table 5.4**).

TABLE 5.4 — Arterial Blood Gas Abnormalities Based on Severity of Asthma

	Asthma Severity			
	I Mild	II Moderate	III Severe	IV Prearrest
PaO_2	Normal	Slight decrease	Moderate decrease	Moderate decrease
$PaCO_2$	Slight decrease	Moderate decrease	Normal	Moderate increase
pH	Slight increase	Moderate increase	Normal	Decrease

Abbreviations: $PaCO_2$, partial pressure of carbon dioxide in arterial gas; PaO_2, partial pressure of arterial oxygen.

SUGGESTED READING

American Thoracic Society. Lung function testing: selection of reference values and interpretative strategies. *Am Rev Respir Dis.* 1991;144:1202-1218.

Christopher KL, Wood RP II, Eckert RC, Blager FB, Raney RA, Souhrada JF. Vocal-cord dysfunction presenting as asthma. *N Engl J Med.* 1983;308:1566-1570.

Clinical Practice Guidelines. Expert Panel Report 2: Guidelines for the Diagnosis and Management of Asthma. Bethesda, Md: US Dept of Health and Human Services, Public Health Service, National Institutes of Health, National Heart, Lung, and Blood Institute; 1997. NIH publication 97-4051.

Corre KA, Rothstein RJ. Assessing severity of adult asthma and need for hospitalization. *Ann Emerg Med.* 1985;14:45-52.

Downing ET, Braman SS, Fox MJ, Corrao WM. Factitious asthma. Physiological approach to diagnosis. *JAMA.* 1982;248:2878-2881.

Expert Panel Report of the National Asthma Education and Prevention Program. Guidelines for the Diagnosis and Management of Asthma. Bethesda, Md: National Institutes of Health; 1991:1-136.

Fischl MA, Pitchenik A, Gardner LB. An index predicting relapse and need for hospitalization in patients with acute bronchial asthma. *N Engl J Med.* 1981;305:783-789.

Jain P, Kavuru MS, Emerman CL, Ahmad M. Utility of peak expiratory flow monitoring. *Chest.* 1998;114:861-876.

Kavuru MS, Eliachar I, Sivak ED. Management of the upper airway in the critically ill patient. In: Sivak ED, Higgins T, Seiver A, eds. *The High Risk Patient*: *Management of the Critically Ill.* Baltimore, Md: Williams & Wilkins; 1995:189-211.

McFadden ER Jr, Kiser R, DeGroot WJ. Acute bronchial asthma. Relations between clinical and physiologic manifestations. *N Engl J Med.* 1973;288:221-225.

McFadden ER Jr, Lyons HA. Arterial-blood gas tension in asthma. *N Engl J Med.* 1968;278:1027-1032.

McFadden ER Jr, Zawadski DK. Vocal cord dysfunction masquerading as exercise-induced asthma: a physiologic cause for "choking" during athletic activities. *Am J Respir Crit Care Med*. 1996;153:942-947.

Miller MR, Hankinson J, Brusasco V, et al. Standardisation of spirometry. *Eur Respir J*. 2005;26:319-338.

Miller RD, Hyatt RE. Evaluation of obstructing lesions of the trachea and larynx by flow-volume loops. *Am Rev Respir Dis*. 1973; 108:475-481.

National Heart, Lung, and Blood Institute, National Asthma Education and Prevention Program. Expert panel report 3: guidelines for the diagnosis and management of asthma. August 28, 2007. http://www.nhlbi.nih.gov/guidelines/asthma/asthgdln.pdf. Accessed November 1, 2007.

Nowak RM, Tomlanovich MC, Sarkar DD, Kvale PA, Anderson JA. Arterial blood gases and pulmonary function testing in acute bronchial asthma. Predicting patient outcomes. *JAMA*. 1983;249: 2043-2046.

6

Nonpharmacologic Therapy

Goals and Key Components of Asthma Therapy

The general goals of asthma therapy are outlined in **Table 6**.1. Overall, asthma therapy has four key components (**Table 6**.2).

The National Asthma Education and Prevention Program Expert Panel Report (EPR-3) guidelines target therapy based on the severity of asthma (**Figures 5**.1, **5**.2, **5**.3, **7**.1, **7**.2, and **7**.3).

Nonpharmacologic therapy for chronic asthma begins with the assessment of lung function and disease severity and is discussed in Chapter 5, *Clinical Evaluation and Assessment of Severity*.

Additionally, the EPR-3 suggests that patient education and self-management and the environmental control and avoidance of asthma triggers may play an important role in maintenance therapy of chronic asthma.

Patient Education

Asthma self-management education has received increasing attention in the literature. A number of recent studies have highlighted the beneficial effects as well as the limitations of adult asthma education in clinical practice. The programs have typically involved a combination of widely accepted modalities, including vigorous education about:

- Self-management skills
- A written crisis plan
- Easy access to a nurse practitioner

TABLE 6.1 — Goals of Asthma Therapy

- Prevent chronic and troublesome symptoms
- Maintain near-normal pulmonary function
- Maintain normal activity levels, including exercise and other physical activity
- Prevent recurrent exacerbations of asthma and minimize the need for emergency department visits or hospitalizations
- Provide optimal pharmacotherapy with minimal or no adverse effects
- Meet patients' and families' expectations of satisfaction with asthma care

Clinical Practice Guidelines. Expert Panel Report 2: Guidelines for the Diagnosis and Management of Asthma. Bethesda, Md: US Dept of Health and Human Services; 1997. NIH publication 97-4051.

TABLE 6.2 — Four Key Components of Asthma Therapy

- Patient education and self-management
- Objective assessment of lung function and disease severity, including home PEF monitoring
- Environmental control with avoidance of asthma triggers
- Pharmacologic therapy

Abbreviation: PEF, peak expiratory flow.

- Home peak expiratory flow (PEF) monitoring
- Proper metered-dose inhaler (MDI) technique (see Chapter 8, *Bronchodilators*).

The EPR-2 recommends that patients, especially those with moderate-to-severe persistent asthma or a history of severe exacerbations, be given a written action plan based on signs and symptoms and/or PEF. Some programs have resulted in a 3-fold reduction in readmission rate and a 2-fold reduction in hospital day-use rate.

Specifically, small group and individual asthma education programs improve:

- Patient understanding
- The ability to control asthma symptoms
- MDI technique.

Additional controlled studies involving formal asthma education programs have documented their effectiveness in reducing the use of health services. Other studies have documented the cost effectiveness of an adult asthma education program. However, attendance rates for formal asthma education programs have ranged from 31% to 66%. Attendees at asthma education programs were more likely to be:

- Women
- Nonsmokers
- Patients from a higher socioeconomic status.

Peak Expiratory Flow Monitoring

Peak expiratory flow monitoring has been advocated as an objective measure of airflow obstruction in patients with chronic asthma. All published asthma practice guidelines uniformly recommend the use of PEF monitoring as an adjunct to asthma education in selected groups of patients. Unfortunately, even after nearly 4 decades of use, many aspects of PEF monitoring remain unclear. An important and largely unanswered question is whether PEF monitoring adds anything to a well-constructed, individualized asthma education program with management based on symptoms alone. Despite a sound theoretic rationale for PEF monitoring, clinical trials that studied the usefulness of PEF monitoring in ambulatory asthma patients show conflicting results. Over the past decade, six out of ten randomized trials failed to show an advantage for the addition of PEF monitoring above and beyond symptom-based intervention for the control group.

Although PEF monitoring is not an adequate substitute for office spirometry in the initial diagnosis, currently available inexpensive devices are acceptable for serial monitoring of airflow obstruction. Irrespective of the device used, regular PEF monitoring allows early detection of worsening airflow obstruction, which may be of particular value in "poor perceivers." Even though additional benefits above a well-constructed, symptom-based management plan have not been shown in patients with mild asthma, available data appear to support its role in moderate-to-severe asthma. PEF monitoring has some value in risk-stratification in patients with asthma. Excessive diurnal variation and morning dip of PEF imply poor control and need for careful reevaluation of the management plan. PEF alone is never appropriate; rather, PEF should be part of a comprehensive patient education program. Future studies to evaluate the usefulness of PEF should target patients who are at higher risk for asthma-related morbidity and mortality. These are patients who are suspected to be poor perceivers. Future studies also need to identify the cutoff points or "action points" of high discriminatory value that can be easily applied by both patients and physicians in a primary care setting.

Control of Factors Contributing to Asthma Severity

A variety of population and clinical studies have strongly suggested that exposure to aeroallergens in a susceptible host is associated with allergic sensitization in a subset of patients with both acute and chronic asthma. It is generally accepted that environmental control measures to reduce exposure to allergens should be considered in most asthmatics and immunotherapy should be reserved for selected patients only.

Broadly speaking, aeroallergens can be divided into outdoor allergens (pollen and molds) and indoor allergens (house dust mites, animal allergens, cockroach allergen and indoor molds). Exposure to outdoor allergens is best reduced during the peak pollen season by remaining indoors, in a climate-controlled environment with the windows closed as much as possible.

Much attention in the literature has recently focused on the composition of house dust and indoor allergens. It appears that house dust itself is not an allergen, but there are allergic components within house dust. Fecal pellets from two house dust mites, *Dermatophagoides farinae* and *D. pteronyssinus*, contain several well-characterized allergens (*Der f I*, *Der f II*, *Der p I*, and *Der p II*). Similarly, allergens from cat dander (*Fel d I*) and cockroaches (*Bla g I*, *Bla g II*) have been well described.

Data suggest that certain environmental conditions such as high temperature, humidity, and perhaps closed urban surroundings can increase allergen burden from these sources. A variety of studies have quantitatively measured these allergens and have recommended safe levels. Specific recommendations have been published to help reduce indoor allergen burden. Overall, it seems clear that indoor allergens contribute to some morbidity related to asthma and that strategies to minimize allergen exposure are warranted in most asthma patients.

The key points of controlling factors that contribute to asthma are outlined in **Table 6.3**. Skin testing or *in vitro* testing is now specifically recommended for at least those patients with persistent asthma who are exposed to perennial indoor allergens. Routine use of chemicals to kill house dust mites and denature the antigen is no longer recommended as a control measure. Annual influenza vaccinations are now specifically recommended for patients with persistent asthma. Adult patients with severe persistent asthma, nasal polyps, or a history of sensitivity to aspirin or nonsteroidal anti-inflammatory agents are to be

TABLE 6.3 — Control of Factors Contributing to Asthma Severity

- Exposure of asthma patients to irritants or allergens to which they are sensitive has been shown to increase asthma symptoms and precipitate asthma exacerbations.
- For at least those patients with persistent asthma who are on daily medications, the clinician should:
  - Identify allergen exposures
  - Use the patient's history to assess sensitivity to seasonal allergens
  - Use skin testing or *in vitro* testing to assess sensitivity to perennial indoor allergens
  - Assess the significance of positive tests in context of patients' medical history.
- Patients with asthma at any level of severity should avoid:
  - Exposure to allergens to which they are sensitive
  - Exposure to environmental tobacco smoke
  - Exertion when levels of air pollution are high
  - Use of β-blockers
  - Sulfite-containing and other foods to which they are sensitive.
- Adult patients should be counseled regarding the risk of severe and even fatal exacerbations from using these drugs if they have:
  - Severe persistent asthma
  - Nasal polyps
  - A history of sensitivity to aspirin or nonsteroidal anti-inflammatory agents.
- Patients should be treated for rhinitis, sinusitis, and gastroesophageal reflux, if present.
- Patients with persistent asthma should be given an annual influenza vaccine.

counseled regarding the risk of severe and even fatal exacerbations from using these drugs.

For successful long-term asthma management, it is essential to identify and reduce exposures to relevant allergens and irritants and to control other factors that have been shown to increase asthma symptoms and/or precipitate asthma exacerbations. These factors fall into four categories:

- Inhalant allergens:
  - Animal allergens
  - House dust mites
  - Cockroach allergens
  - Indoor fungi (molds)
  - Outdoor allergens
- Occupational exposures:
  - Tobacco smoke
  - Indoor/outdoor pollution and irritants
- Nonallergic factors
- Other factors:
  - Rhinitis/sinusitis
  - Gastroesophageal reflux
  - Sensitivity to aspirin, other nonsteroid anti-inflammatory drugs, and sulfites
  - Ophthalmic and systemic β-blockers
  - Viral respiratory infections.

SUGGESTED READING

Allergen Avoidance

Busse PJ, Wang JJ, Halm EA. Allergen sensitization evaluation and allergen avoidance education in an inner-city adult cohort with persistent asthma. *J Allergy Clin Immunol.* 2005;116:146-152.

Call RS, Smith TF, Morris E, Chapman MD, Platts-Mills TA. Risk factors for asthma in inner city children. *J Pediatr.* 1992;121:862-866.

Creticos PS. Immunotherapy with allergens. *JAMA.* 1992;268:2834-2839.

Creticos PS, Reed CE, Norman PS, et al. Ragweed immunotherapy in adult asthma. *N Engl J Med*. 1996;334:501-506.

Gelber LE, Seltzer LH, Bouzoukis JK, Pollart SM, Chapman MD, Platts-Mills TA. Sensitization and exposure to indoor allergens as risk factors for asthma among patients presenting to hospital. *Am Rev Respir Dis*. 1993;147:573-578.

Hamilton RG, Chapman MD, Platts-Mills TA, Adkinson NF. House dust aeroallergen measurements in clinical practice: a guide to allergen-free home and work environments. *Immunol Allergy Pract*. 1992;14:96-112.

Platts-Mills TA. Allergen-specific treatment for asthma: III. *Am Rev Respir Dis*. 1993;148:553-555. Editorial.

Platts-Mills TA, de Weck AL. Dust mite allergens and asthma – a worldwide problem. *J Allergy Clin Immunol*. 1989;83:416-427.

Sporik R, Holgate ST, Platts-Mills TA, Cogswell JJ. Exposure to house-dust mite allergen (*Der p I*) and the development of asthma in childhood. A prospective study. *N Engl J Med*. 1990;323:502-507.

Patient Education

Bailey WC, Richards JM Jr, Brooks CM, Soong SJ, Windsor RA, Manzella BA. A randomized trial to improve self-management practices of adults with asthma. *Arch Intern Med*. 1990;150:1664-1668.

Bolton MB, Tilley BC, Kuder J, Reeves T, Schultz LR. The cost and effectiveness of an education program for adults who have asthma. *J Gen Intern Med*. 1991;6:401-407.

Cabana MD, Le TT. Challenges in asthma patient education. *J Allergy Clin Immunol*. 2005;115:1225-1227.

Clark NM. Asthma self-management education. Research and implications for clinical practice. *Chest*. 1989;95:1110-1113.

Clark NM, Feldman CH, Evans D, Levison MJ, Wasilewski Y, Mellins RB. The impact of health education on frequency and cost of health care use by low income children with asthma. *J Allergy Clin Immunol*. 1986;78:108-115.

Hilton S, Sibbald B, Anderson HR, Freeling P. Controlled evaluation of the effects of patient education on asthma morbidity in general practice. *Lancet*. 1986;1:26-29.

Mayo PH, Richman J, Harris HW. Results of a program to reduce admissions for adult asthma. *Ann Intern Med.* 1990;112:864-871.

Parker SR, Mellins RB, Sogn DD. NHBLI workshop summary. Asthma education: a national strategy. *Am Rev Respir Dis.* 1989; 140:848-853.

Tougaard L, Krone T, Sorknaes A, Ellegaard H. Economic benefits of teaching patients with chronic obstructive pulmonary disease about their illness. *Lancet.* 1992;339:1517-1520.

Wilson SR, Scamagas P, German DF, et al. A controlled trial of two forms of self-management education for adults with asthma. *Am J Med.* 1993;94:564-576.

Yoon R, McKenzie DK, Miles DA, Bauman A. Characteristics of attenders and non-attenders at an asthma education programme. *Thorax.* 1991;46:886-890.

6

Peak Expiratory Flow Monitoring

Cote J, Cartier A, Robichaud P, et al. Influence on asthma morbidity of asthma education programs based on self-management plans following treatment optimization. *Am J Respir Crit Care Med.* 1997;155:1509-1514.

Cowie RL, Revitt SG, Underwood MF, Field SK. The effect of a peak flow-based action plan in the prevention of exacerbations of asthma. *Chest.* 1997;112:1534-1538.

Jain P, Kavuru MS, Emerman CL, Ahmad M. Utility of peak expiratory flow monitoring. *Chest.* 1998;114:861-876.

Turner MO, Taylor D, Bennett R, Fitzgerald JM. A randomized trial comparing peak expiratory flow and symptom self-management plans for patients with asthma attending a primary care clinic. *Am J Respir Crit Care Med.* 1998;157:540-546.

7
Overview of Pharmacologic Management

Pharmacotherapy for Asthma

The pharmacotherapy for asthma can be classified as:

- Quick relief or symptomatic therapy with bronchodilators:
  - β-Agonists
  - Theophylline
- Long-term control with anti-inflammatory agents:
  - Corticosteroids
  - Cromolyn sodium
  - Nedocromil sodium
  - Antileukotrienes
  - Monoclonal anti-IgE antibodies.

For a summary of mechanisms of action for available asthma medications, see **Table 7.1**. These pharmacologic classes of pharmacologic agents are discussed in more detail in subsequent chapters.

Management Guidelines

The National Asthma Education and Prevention Program (NAEPP) *Expert Panel Report 3 (EPR-3): Guidelines for the Diagnosis and Management of Asthma* updated selected recommendations of the previous Expert Panel Report, published in 2002. Both of these guidelines provide an excellent algorithmic framework for the management of bronchial asthma.

TABLE 7.1 — Mechanisms of Action of Available Asthma Medications

β-Agonist
- Stimulates β_2-receptors
- Activates adenylate cyclase; increases intracellular cyclic adenosine monophosphate (cAMP)
- Affects compartmental shifts in calcium
- Directs bronchial smooth muscle relaxation
- ? Decreases mediator release from mast cells

Methylxanthine
- Directs relaxation of bronchial smooth muscle (? mechanism)
- Inhibits mast cell degranulation
- Antagonizes effects of adenosine on mast cells, reducing mediator release
- Improves macociliary transport, diaphragm contractility

Corticosteroid
- Reduces number of mucosal mast cells
- Enhances β-adrenergic receptor sensitivity
- Produces phospholipase A_2-inhibitors
- Suppresses various late-phase inflammatory reactions

Cromolyn Sodium
- Stablize mast cells
- Affects mast cell calcium channels
- Phosphorylates membrane proteins needed for degranulation process
- ? Other late phase effects

Nedocromil Sodium
- Supresses various early- and late-phase inflammatory reactions
- Inhibits eosinophils, mast cells, platelets, neutrophils
- Inhibits airway axonal reflexes
- Prevents stimulation of C fibers (antitussive effect)

Antileukotriene
- Antagonizes cysteinyl leukotriene (cys-LT_1 or LTD_4) receptors
- Inhibits 5-lipoxygenase

Anti-IgE Monoclonal Antibodies
- Selectively bind free (not receptor-bound) IgE
- Reduce serum levels of IgE

According to the most recent guidelines, the goals of therapy for asthma control are:

- Minimal or no chronic day or night symptoms
- Minimal or no exacerbations
- Maintain (near) normal pulmonary function (adults/children >5 years of age)
- No limitations on activities: no school/work (or parent work) missed
- Minimal use of short-acting inhaled β_2-agonists
- Minimal or no adverse effects from medications

■ Stepwise Approach to Pharmacologic Management

The 2002 and 2007 NAEPP guidelines recommend a stepwise approach to the pharmacologic management of asthma that is based on classification of the severity of the patient's symptoms, level of asthma control achieved, and other clinical findings (eg, pulmonary function):

- Treatment should be based on the most severe step in which any clinical feature occurs.
- Treatment should be reviewed every 1 to 6 months; a gradual stepwise reduction in treatment may be possible.
- If control is not maintained, step-up should be considered. However, the patient's medication technique, adherence, and environmental control should first be reviewed.

The recommended stepwise approach for outpatient management of acute or chronic asthma in children 0 to 4 years of age is shown in **Figure 7.1**, for children 5 to 11 years of age is shown in **Figure 7.2**, and the stepwise approach in adults and youths ≥12 years of age is shown in **Figure 7.3**.

An algorithm for the home management of acute exacerbations of asthma in adults is shown in **Figure**

FIGURE 7.1 — Stepwise Approach for Managing Asthma in Children 0 to 4 Years of Age

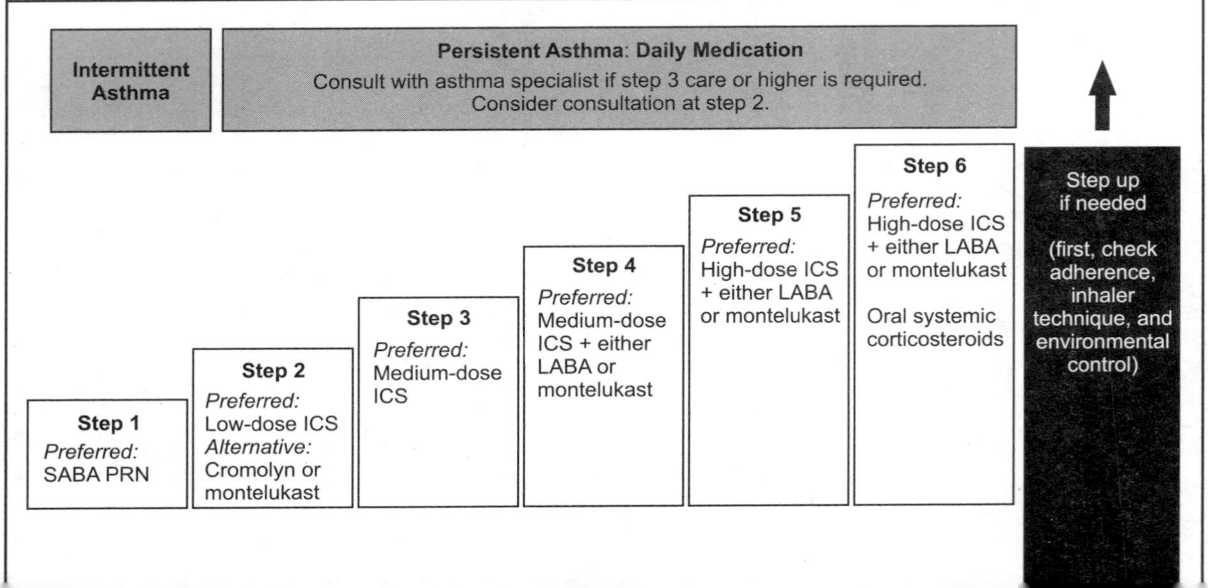

Intermittent Asthma	Persistent Asthma: Daily Medication
	Consult with asthma specialist if step 3 care or higher is required. Consider consultation at step 2.

Step 1
Preferred:
SABA PRN

Step 2
Preferred:
Low-dose ICS
Alternative:
Cromolyn or montelukast

Step 3
Preferred:
Medium-dose ICS

Step 4
Preferred:
Medium-dose ICS + either LABA or montelukast

Step 5
Preferred:
High-dose ICS + either LABA or montelukast

Step 6
Preferred:
High-dose ICS + either LABA or montelukast
Oral systemic corticosteroids

→ Step up if needed
(first, check adherence, inhaler technique, and environmental control)

Step down if possible

(and asthma is well controlled at least 3 months)

Patient Education and Environmental Control at Each Step

Quick-Relief Medication for All Patients
- SABA as needed for symptoms. Intensity of treatment depends on severity of symptoms.
- With viral respiratory infection: SABA q 4-6 hours up to 24 hours (longer with physician consult). Consider short course of oral systemic corticosteroids if exacerbation is severe or patient has history of previous severe exacerbations.
- Caution: Frequent use of SABA may indicate the need to step up treatment. See text for recommendations on initiating daily long-term–control therapy.

Abbreviations: ICS, inhaled corticosteroid; LABA, inhaled long-acting β₂-agonist; PRN, as required; q, every; SABA, inhaled short-acting β₂-agonist.

- The stepwise approach is meant to assist, not replace, the clinical decision making required to meet individual patient needs.
- If alternative treatment is used and response is inadequate, discontinue it and use the preferred treatment before stepping up.
- If clear benefit is not observed within 4 to 6 weeks and patient/family medication technique and adherence are satisfactory, consider adjusting therapy or alternative diagnosis.
- Studies on children 0 to 4 years of age are limited. Step 2 preferred therapy is based on Evidence A. All other recommendations are based on expert opinion and extrapolation from studies in older children.

National Heart, Lung, and Blood Institute. National Asthma Education and Prevention Program. *Expert panel report 3: guidelines for the diagnosis and management of asthma;* August 28, 2007. *http://www.nhlbi.nih.gov/guidelines/asthma/asthgdln.pdf.* Accessed November 1, 2007.

7

FIGURE 7.2 — Stepwise Approach for Managing Asthma in Children 5 to 11 Years of Age

Intermittent Asthma

Persistent Asthma: Daily Medication
Consult with asthma specialist if step 4 care or higher is required.
Consider consultation at step 3.

Step 1
Preferred:
SABA PRN

Step 2
Preferred:
Low-dose ICS

Alternative:
Cromolyn,
LTRA,
nedocromil, or
theophylline

Step 3
Preferred:
EITHER:
Low-dose ICS
+ either LABA,
LTRA, or
theophylline
OR
Medium-dose
ICS

Step 4
Preferred:
Medium-dose
ICS + LABA

Alternative:
Medium-dose
ICS + either
LTRA or
theophylline

Step 5
Preferred:
High-dose ICS
+ LABA

Alternative:
High-dose ICS
+ either LTRA
or theophylline

Step 6
Preferred:
High-dose ICS
+ LABA + oral
systemic
corticosteroid

Alternative:
High-dose ICS
+ either LTRA
or theophylline
+ oral systemic
corticosteroid

Step up
if needed

(first, check
adherence,
inhaler
technique,
environmental
control, and
comorbid
conditions)

Step down if possible

(and asthma is well controlled at least 3 months)

Patient Education, Environmental Control, and Management of Comorbidities at Each Step
Steps 2-4: Consider SC allergen immunotherapy for patients who have allergic asthma (see legend).

Quick-Relief Medication for All Patients
- SABA as needed for symptoms. Intensity of treatment depends on severity of symptoms: up to 3 treatments at 20-minute intervals as needed. Short course of oral systemic corticosteroids may be needed.
- Caution: Increasing use of SABA or use >2 days a week for symptom relief (not prevention of EIB) generally indicates inadequate control and the need to step up treatment.

Abbreviations: ICS, inhaled corticosteroid; LABA, inhaled long-acting β_2-agonist; LTRA, leukotriene receptor antagonist; PRN, as required; SABA, inhaled short-acting β_2-agonist; SC, subcutaneous.

- The stepwise approach is meant to assist, not replace, the clinical decision making required to meet individual patient needs.
- If alternative treatment is used and response is inadequate, discontinue it and use the preferred treatment before stepping up.
- Theophylline is a less desirable alternative due to the need to monitor serum concentration levels.
- Step 1 and step 2 medications are based on Evidence A. Step 3 ICS + adjunctive therapy and ICS are based on Evidence B for efficacy of each treatment and extrapolation from comparator trials in older children and adults—comparator trials are not available for this age group; steps 4 through 6 are based on expert opinion and extrapolation from studies in older children and adults.
- Immunotherapy for steps 2 through 4 is based on Evidence B for house-dust mites, animal danders, and pollens; evidence is weak or lacking for molds and cockroaches. Evidence is strongest for immunotherapy with single allergens. The role of allergy in asthma is greater in children than in adults. Clinicians who administer immunotherapy should be prepared and equipped to identify and treat anaphylaxis that may occur.

National Heart, Lung, and Blood Institute. National Asthma Education and Prevention Program. *Expert panel report 3: guidelines for the diagnosis and management of asthma*; August 28, 2007. *http://www.nhlbi.nih.gov/guidelines/asthma/asthgdln.pdf*. Accessed November 1, 2007.

7

FIGURE 7.3 — Stepwise Approach for Managing Asthma in Youths ≥12 Years of Age and Adults

Intermittent Asthma

Persistent Asthma: Daily Medication
Consult with asthma specialist if step 4 care or higher is required.
Consider consultation at step 3.

Step up if needed
(first, check adherence, environmental control, and comorbid conditions)

Step 1
Preferred:
SABA PRN

Step 2
Preferred:
Low-dose ICS

Alternative:
Cromolyn, LTRA, nedocromil, or theophylline

Step 3
Preferred:
Low-dose ICS + LABA or medium-dose ICS

Alternative:
Low-dose ICS + either LTRA, theophylline, or zileuton

Step 4
Preferred:
Medium-dose ICS + LABA

Alternative:
Medium-dose ICS + either LTRA, theophylline, or zileuton

Step 5
Preferred:
High-dose ICS + LABA

AND

Consider omalizumab for patients who have allergies

Step 6
Preferred:
High-dose ICS + LABA + oral systemic corticosteroids

AND

Consider omalizumab for patients who have allergies

Step down if possible

(and asthma is well controlled at least 3 months)

Patient Education, Environmental Control, and Management of Comorbidities at Each Step

Steps 2-4: Consider SC allergen immunotherapy for patients who have allergic asthma (see legend).

Quick-Relief Medication for All Patients

- SABA as needed for symptoms. Intensity of treatment depends on severity of symptoms: up to 3 treatments at 20-minute intervals as needed. Short course of oral systemic corticosteroids may be needed.
- Use of SABA >2 days a week for symptom relief (not prevention of EIB) generally indicates inadequate control and the need to step up treatment.

Abbreviations: EIB, exercise-induced bronchospasm; EPR, Expert Panel Report; ICS, inhaled corticosteroid; LABA, inhaled long-acting β_2-agonist; LTRA, leukotriene receptor antagonist; PRN, as required; SABA, inhaled short-acting β_2-agonist; SC, subcutaneous.

- The stepwise approach is meant to assist, not replace, the clinical decision making required to meet individual patient needs.
- If alternative treatment is used and response is inadequate, discontinue it and use the preferred treatment before stepping up.
- Zileuton is a less desirable alternative due to limited studies as adjunctive therapy and the need to monitor liver function. Theophylline requires monitoring of serum concentration levels.
- In step 6, before oral systemic corticosteroids are introduced, a trial of high-dose ICS + LABA + either LTRA, theophylline, or zileuton may be considered, although this approach has not been studied in clinical trials.
- Step 1, 2, and 3 preferred therapies are based on Evidence A; step 3 alternative therapy is based on Evidence A for LTRA, Evidence B for theophylline, and Evidence D for zileuton. Step 4 preferred therapy is based on Evidence B, and alternative therapy is based on Evidence B for LTRA and theophylline and Evidence D for zileuton. Step 5 preferred therapy is based on Evidence B. Step 6 preferred therapy is based on (EPR—2 1997) and Evidence B for omalizumab.

7

Continued

79

- Immunotherapy for steps 2 through 4 is based on Evidence B for house-dust mites, animal danders, and pollens; evidence is weak or lacking for molds and cockroaches. Evidence is strongest for immunotherapy with single allergens. The role of allergy in asthma is greater in children than in adults.
- Clinicians who administer immunotherapy or omalizumab should be prepared and equipped to identify and treat anaphylaxis that may occur.

National Heart, Lung, and Blood Institute. National Asthma Education and Prevention Program. *Expert panel report 3: guidelines for the diagnosis and management of asthma;* August 28, 2007. *http://www.nhlbi.nih.gov/guidelines/asthma/asthgdln.pdf.* Accessed November 1, 2007.

7.4, while algorithms for emergency department and hospital-based care are shown in **Figure 7.5**.

Key general recommendations are also provided for managing asthma in different patient populations, namely:

- In infants and young children:
  - Diagnosing asthma in infants is often difficult, yet underdiagnosis and undertreatment are key problems in this age group. Thus a diagnostic trial of inhaled bronchodilators and anti-inflammatory medications may be helpful.
  - In general, infants and young children consistently requiring symptomatic treatment more than two times per week should be given daily anti-inflammatory therapy.
  - When initiating daily anti-inflammatory therapy, a trial of cromolyn sodium or nedocromil sodium is often given due to the safety profile of these medications.
  - Response to therapy should be carefully monitored. Once control of asthma symptoms is established and sustained, a careful step-down in therapy should be attempted. If clear benefit is not observed, alternative therapies or diagnoses should be considered.
- In school-age children and adolescents:
  - Pulmonary function testing should use appropriate reference populations. Predicted norms of adolescents compare better with those of childhood than with those of adults.
  - When initiating daily anti-inflammatory therapy for mild-to-moderate persistent asthma, a trial of cromolyn sodium or nedocromil sodium is often given.
  - Adolescents (and younger children as appropriate) should be directly involved in

FIGURE 7.4 — Management of Asthma Exacerbations: Home Treatment

Assess Severity

- Patients at high risk for a fatal attack require immediate medical attention after initial treatment
- Symptoms and signs suggestive of a more serious exacerbation such as marked breathlessness, inability to speak more than short phrases, use of accessory muscles, or drowsiness should result in initial treatment while immediately consulting with a clinician
- Less severe signs and symptoms can be treated initially with assessment of response to therapy and further steps as listed below
- If available, measure PEF—values of 50% to 79% predicted or personal best indicate the need for quick-relief mediation. Depending on the response to treatment, contact with a clinician may also be indicated. Values below 50% indicate the need for immediate medical care

Initial Treatment

- Inhaled SABA: up to two treatments 20 minutes part of 2 to 6 puffs by MDI or nebulizer treatments
- Note: Medication delivery is highly variable. Children and individuals who have exacerbations of lesser severity may need fewer puffs than suggested above

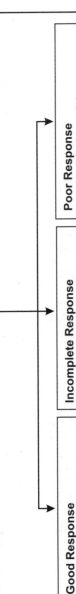

Good Response
No wheezing or dyspnea (assess tachypnea in young children)
PEF ≥80% predicted or personal best

- Contact clinician for follow-up instructions and further management
- May continue inhaled SABA every 3 to 4 hours for 24 to 48 hours
- Consider short course of oral systemic corticosteroids

Incomplete Response
Persistent wheezing and dyspnea (tachypnea)
PEF 50% to 79% predicted or personal best

- Add oral systemic corticosteroid
- Continue inhaled SABA
- Contact clinician urgently (this day) for further instruction

To ED

Poor Response
Marked wheezing and dyspnea
PEF <50% predicted or personal best

- Add oral systemic corticosteroid
- Repeat inhaled SABA immediately
- If distress is severe and nonresponsive to initial treatment:
  – Call your doctor AND
  – **PROCEED TO ED**
  – Consider calling 9-1-1 (ambulance transport)

Abbreviations: ED, emergency department; MDI, metered-dose inhaler; PEF, peak expiratory flow; SABA, short-acting β_2-agonist (quick-relief inhaler).

National Heart, Lung, and Blood Institute. National Asthma Education and Prevention Program. *Expert panel report 3: guidelines for the diagnosis and management of asthma*; August 28, 2007. http://www.nhlbi.nih.gov/guidelines/asthma/asthgdln.pdf. Accessed November 1, 2007.

FIGURE 7.5 — Management of Asthma Exacerbations: ED and Hospital-Based Care

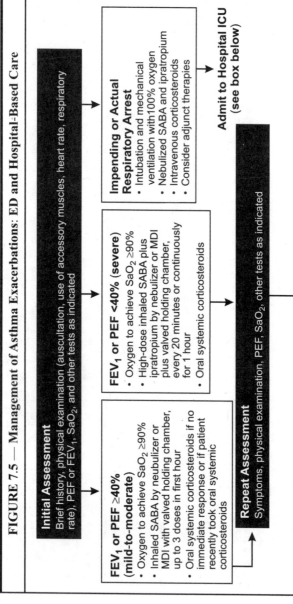

Initial Assessment

Brief history, physical examination (auscultation, use of accessory muscles, heart rate, respiratory rate), PEF or FEV$_1$, SaO$_2$, and other tests as indicated

FEV$_1$ or PEF ≥40% (mild-to-moderate)
- Oxygen to achieve SaO$_2$ ≥90%
- Inhaled SABA by neubulizer or MDI with valved holding chamber, up to 3 doses in first hour
- Oral systemic corticosteroids if no immediate response or if patient recently took oral systemic corticosteroids

FEV$_1$ or PEF <40% (severe)
- Oxygen to achieve SaO$_2$ ≥90%
- High-dose inhaled SABA plus ipratropium by nebulizer or MDI plus valved holding chamber, every 20 minutes or continuously for 1 hour
- Oral systemic corticosteroids

Impending or Actual Respiratory Arrest
- Intubation and mechanical ventilation with 100% oxygen
- Nebulized SABA and ipratropium
- Intravenous corticosteroids
- Consider adjunct therapies

Admit to Hospital ICU (see box below)

Repeat Assessment

Symptoms, physical examination, PEF, SaO$_2$, other tests as indicated

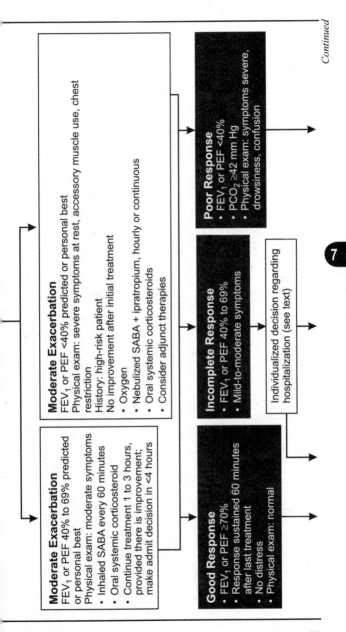

Moderate Exacerbation
FEV$_1$ or PEF 40% to 69% predicted
or personal best
Physical exam: moderate symptoms
- Inhaled SABA every 60 minutes
- Oral systemic corticosteroid
- Continue treatment 1 to 3 hours, provided there is improvement; make admit decision in <4 hours

Moderate Exacerbation
FEV$_1$ or PEF <40% predicted or personal best
Physical exam: severe symptoms at rest, accessory muscle use, chest restriction
History: high-risk patient
No improvement after initial treatment
- Oxygen
- Nebulized SABA + ipratropium, hourly or continuous
- Oral systemic corticosteroids
- Consider adjunct therapies

Good Response
- FEV$_1$ or PEF ≥70%
- Response sustained 60 minutes after last treatment
- No distress
- Physical exam: normal

Incomplete Response
- FEV$_1$ or PEF 40% to 69%
- Mild-to-moderate symptoms

Poor Response
- FEV$_1$ or PEF <40%
- PCO$_2$ ≥42 mm Hg
- Physical exam: symptoms severe, drowsiness, confusion

Individualized decision regarding hospitalization (see text)

Continued

7

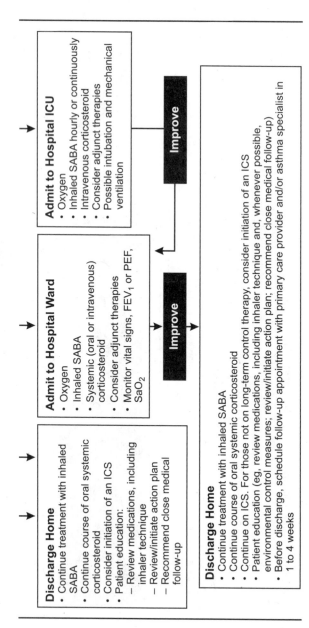

Discharge Home
- Continue treatment with inhaled SABA
- Continue course of oral systemic corticosteroid
- Consider initiation of an ICS
- Patient education:
  - Review medications, including inhaler technique
  - Review/initiate action plan
  - Recommend close medical follow-up

Admit to Hospital Ward
- Oxygen
- Inhaled SABA
- Systemic (oral or intravenous) corticosteroid
- Consider adjunct therapies
- Monitor vital signs, FEV_1 or PEF, SaO_2

Improve

Admit to Hospital ICU
- Oxygen
- Inhaled SABA hourly or continuously
- Intravenous corticosteroid
- Consider adjunct therapies
- Possible intubation and mechanical ventilation

Improve

Discharge Home
- Continue treatment with inhaled SABA
- Continue course of oral systemic corticosteroid
- Continue on ICS. For those not on long-term control therapy, consider initiation of an ICS
- Patient education (eg, review medications, including inhaler technique and, whenever possible, environmental control measures; review/initiate action plan; recommend close medical follow-up)
- Before discharge, schedule follow-up appointment with primary care provider and/or asthma specialist in 1 to 4 weeks

Abbreviations: ED, emergency department; FEV_1, forced expiratory volume in 1 second; ICS, inhaled corticosteroids; MDI, metered-dose inhaler; PCO_2, partial pressure carbon dioxide; PEF, peak expiratory flow; SABA, short-acting β_2-agonist; SaO_2, oxygen saturation.

National Heart, Lung, and Blood Institute. National Asthma Education and Prevention Program. *Expert panel report 3: guidelines for the diagnosis and management of asthma;* August 28, 2007. *http://www.nhlbi.nih.gov/guidelines/asthma/asthgdln.pdf.* Accessed November 1, 2007.

7

establishing goals for therapy and developing their asthma management plans.

- Active participation in physical activities, exercise, and sports should be promoted.
- A written asthma management plan should be prepared for the student's school, including plans to ensure reliable, prompt access to medications.

• In older adults:

- Chronic bronchitis/emphysema may coexist with asthma. A trial of systemic corticosteroids will determine the presence of reversibility and the extent of therapeutic benefit.
- Asthma medications may aggravate coexisting medical conditions (eg, cardiac disease, osteoporosis); adjustments in the medication plan may need to be made.
- Be aware of increased potential for adverse drug/disease interaction (eg, aspirin, β-blockers).
- Review of patient technique in using medications and devices is essential.

SUGGESTED READING

Expert Panel Report: Guidelines for the Diagnosis and Management of Asthma—Update on Selected Topics 2002. Bethesda, Md: US Dept of Health and Human Services, National Institutes of Health, National Heart, Lung, and Blood Institute, National Asthma Education and Prevention Program; 2003. NIH publication 02-5074.

National Heart, Lung, and Blood Institute, National Asthma Education and Prevention Program. Expert panel report 3: guidelines for the diagnosis and management of asthma. August 28, 2007. http://www.nhlbi.nih.gov/guidelines/asthma/asthgdln.pdf. Accessed November 1, 2007.

8 Bronchodilators

In the United States, there are three major classes of sympathomimetic bronchodilators available:

- *Catecholamines*:
  - Examples include:
    - Isoproterenol
    - Isoetharine
  - Are rapid-acting
  - Are potent
  - Are relatively nonselective β_1-agonists
- *Resorcinols*:
  - Examples include:
    - Metaproterenol
    - Terbutaline
  - Represent a modification of the catechol nucleus, resulting in a long-acting drug that is relatively β_2-selective, this selectivity being dose-dependent
- *Saligenins*:
  - Examples include:
    - Albuterol
    - Formoterol
  - Salmeterol
  - Represent a modification of the catechol nucleus, resulting in a long-acting drug that is relatively β_2-selective.

Mechanism of Action and Pharmacology of Bronchodilators

The sympathomimetics activate adenylate cyclase and thereby increase intracellular cyclic adenosine monophosphate (cAMP). This, in turn, provides energy for compartmental shifts in calcium that result in bronchial smooth muscle relaxation.

The major therapeutic actions of β-stimulation in the treatment of asthma include:

- Bronchodilation
- Facilitation of mucociliary clearance.

β-Agonists inhibit acute mediator release from mast cells but do not have an effect on cellular inflammation or the late asthmatic response (LAR).

The pharmacologic effects and pharmacokinetic properties of sympathomimetic bronchodilators are shown in **Table 8.1**. Currently available sympathomimetic bronchodilators are listed in **Table 8.2**.

Role of β-Agonists in Asthma Management

The benefits of inhaled short-acting β-agonists (eg, albuterol, isoproterenol, metaproterenol) used to treat acute exacerbations of asthma have been well-established. However, many patients who experience more than occasional exacerbations require chronic therapy. According to the National Asthma Education and Prevention Program (NAEPP) guidelines, inhaled corticosteroids (ICSs) are first-line therapy. Despite continuing use of ICSs, many patients continue to experience recurrent symptoms requiring a change in maintenance therapy: either an increase in ICS dose or the addition of a bronchodilator. According to the NAEPP guidelines, the preferred second-line agent is a long-acting β-agonist (LABA) in patients 5 years of age and older and a preferred second-line agent in children 0 to 4 years of age with moderate to severe asthma.

As discussed in more detail in Chapter 11, *Add-On and Combination Therapy*, in patients who remain symptomatic on low to high doses of ICSs, the addition of an LABA (currently salmeterol or formoterol) reduces the rate of exacerbations requiring systemic steroids, and improves lung function, asthma symptoms, and use of rescue short-acting β-agonists. Furthermore, clinical trial evidence has shown that the addition of an LABA to ICSs may be more effective that increasing the dose of ICSs.

Thus β-agonist bronchodilators, both short-acting and long-acting, have a major role in the management of patients with persistent asthma. Nevertheless, several concerns have been raised about chronic, long-term treatment with β-agonists (see *The β-Agonist Controversy*, later in this chapter).

Long-Acting β-Agonists

Salmeterol and formoterol are the currently available LABAs. They are best suited for the following clinical situations:

- As adjunctive therapy in patients with suboptimal asthma control while on low-moderate doses of inhaled steroids (as an alternative to increasing the dose of inhaled steroids).
- Predominantly nocturnal asthma symptoms
- Exercise-induced asthma in patients who exercise regularly (may be preferred over short-acting β-agonists)

Both salmeterol and formoterol are indicated for prophylaxis of exercise-induced asthma. However, it is important to educate patients that these bronchodilators are not to be used for rescue relief of acute asthma symptoms. All patients with symptomatic asthma, including those receiving LABAs, should be prescribed and instructed on the proper use of short-acting β-agonists.

The US Food and Drug Administration (FDA) recently mandated the addition of a warning to the package inserts for all products containing LABAs,

TABLE 8.1 — Sympathomimetic Bronchodilators: Pharmacologic Effects and Pharmacokinetic Properties

Sympathomimetic	Adrenergic Receptor Activity	Route of Administration	Onset (minutes)	Duration (hours)
Albuterol*	$\beta_1 < \beta_2$	Orally	Within 30	4 to 8
		Inhalation†	Within 5	3 to 8
Bitolterol*	$\beta_1 < \beta_2$	Inhalation	3 to 4	5 to ≥8
Ephedrine	$\alpha \sim \beta_1 \sim \beta_2$	Orally	Within 60	3 to 5
		Subcutaneous	>20	≤1
		Intramuscular	10 to 20	≤1
		Intravenous	—	—
Epinephrine	$\alpha \sim \beta_1 \sim \beta_2$	Subcutaneous	5 to 15	1 to 4
		Intramuscular	—	1 to 4
		Inhalation†	1 to 5	1 to 3
Ethylnorepinephrine	$\alpha < \beta_1 \sim \beta_2$	Subcutaneous	5 to 10	1 to 2
		Intramuscular	5 to 10	1 to 2

Formoterol	$\beta_1 < \beta_2$	Inhalation (DPI)	5 to 10	12
Isoetharine*	$\beta_1 < \beta_2$	Inhalation†	Within 5	1 to 3
Isoproterenol	$\beta_1 \sim \beta_2$	Sublingually	≈ 30	1 to 2
		Intravenous	Immediate	< 1
		Inhalation†	2 to 5	0.5 to 2
Metaproterenol*	$\beta_1 < \beta_2$	Orally	≈ 30	4
		Inhalation†	5 to 30	2 to 6
Pirbuterol*	$\beta_1 < \beta_2$	Inhalation	Within 5	5
Salmeterol	$\beta_1 < \beta_2$	Inhalation† (DPI, MDI)	10 to 20	12
Terbutaline*	$\beta_1 < \beta_2$	Orally	30	4 to 8
		Subcutaneous	5 to 15	1.5 to 4
		Inhalation	5 to 30	3 to 6

Abbreviations: DPI, dry-powder inhaler; MDI, metered-dose inhaler.

* These agents all have minor β_1 activity.

† May be administered via aerosol nebulizer, bulb nebulizer, or intermittent positive-pressure breathing (IPPB) administration.

Drug Facts and Comparisons 2002. Facts and Comparisons, A Wolters Kluwer Company, St Louis, MO, 2002.

8

TABLE 8.2 — Sympathomimetic Bronchodilators

Generic Name/Trade Name (Manufacturer)	Available Preparation	Suggested Dosage (Adults)
Albuterol sulfate		
AccuNeb (Dey)	Inhalation solution: 1.25 mg/mL; 0.63 mg/mL	1.25 mg or 0.63 mg 3 or 4 times daily as needed
Albuterol (Dey)	Solution: 0.083%	2.5 mg-10 mg q 6-8 hr
Albuterol (Mylan)	Tablets: 2 mg, 4 mg	2 mg-4 mg tid or qid
ProAir HFA (Ivax)	MDI: 90 mcg/inh	2 inh q 4-6 hr or 1 inh q 4 hr
Proventil (Schering)	MDI: 90 mcg/puff	Acute: 2 puffs q 4-6 hr; Max: 8 puffs/day Prophylaxis: 2 puffs 15 min before exercise
	Inhalation solution: 0.083%	2.5 mg tid to qid by nebulization
Proventil HFA* (Schering)	MDI: 90 mcg/puff	2 puffs q 6 hr
Ventolin HFA (GlaxoSmithKline)	MDI: 90 mcg/puff	Acute: 2 puffs q 4-6 hr Prophylaxis: 2 puffs 15 min before exercise
Volmax (Muro)	Tablets: 4 mg, 8 mg (extended release)	4 mg-8 mg q 12 hr; Max: 32 mg/day in divided doses
VoSpire (Odyssey)	Tablets: 4 mg, 8 mg (extended release)	4 mg-8 mg q 12 hr; Max: 32 mg/day in divided doses

Epinephrine		
EpiPen (Dey)	Injection: 0.3 mg auto-injector	0.3 mg intramuscularly
Formoterol fumarate		
Foradil Aerolizer (Schering)	DPI: 12 mcg/dose	1 puff q 12 hr (morning and evening); Prophylaxis: 1 puff 15 min before exercise
Metaproterenol sulfate		
Alupent (Boehringer Ingelheim)	MDI: 15 mg/1 mL (0.65 mg/puff)	2-3 puffs q 3-4 hr; Max: 12 puffs/day
Metaproterenol (Dey)	Tablets: 10 mg, 20 mg	20 mg tid or qid
Metaproterenol (many)	Inhalation solution: 0.4%, 0.6% vials	1 vial/treatment tid-qid
Pirbuterol acetate		
Maxair Autohaler (Graceway)	MDI: 0.2 mg/puff	1-2 puffs q 4-6 hr; Max: 12 puffs/day
Maxair Inhaler (Graceway)	MDI: 0.2 mg/puff	1-2 puffs q 4-6 hr; Max: 12 puffs/day

Continued

8

Generic Name/Trade Name (Manufacturer)	Available Preparation	Suggested Dosage (Adults)
Salmeterol xinafoate		
Serevent (GlaxoSmithKline)	MDI: 42 mcg/puff	Relief: 2 puffs q 12 hr (morning and evening) Prophylaxis: 2 puffs 30-60 min before exercise
Serevent Diskus (GlaxoSmithKline)	DPI: 50 mcg/dose	1 puff q 12 hr (morning and evening)
Terbutaline sulfate		
Brethine (aaiPharma)	Tablets: 2.5 mg, 5 mg SC injection: 1 mg/mL	2.5 mg-5 mg tid; Max: 15 mg/24 hr 0.25 mg SC, second dose of 0.25 SC may be given if improvement not noted in 15-30 min; Max: 0.5 mg/4 hr

Abbreviations: DPI, dry-powder inhaler; hr, hour; inh, inhalation; MDI, metered-dose inhaler; min, minute; q, every; qid, four times a day; SC, subcutaneous; tid, three times a day.

* HFA, hydrofluoroalkane (nonchlorofluorocarbon [CFC] propellant).

which currently includes salmeterol and formoterol, due to the increased risk of asthma-related death. See below in the section, *The β-Agonist Controversy*, for a discussion of this concern.

■ Salmeterol

Salmeterol xinafoate is a long-acting β_2-agonist for use in the treatment of asthma, and is currently available in a metered-dose inhaler (MDI) (Serevent) and a dry-powder inhaler (DPI) (Serevent Diskus). (See Chapter 12, *Inhalation Devices*, for a discussion and description of commonly used inhalation devices.) Salmeterol has a long lipophilic side chain that confers a long duration of action (12 hours). *In vitro* studies suggest that salmeterol is more potent than albuterol and has a slower onset. Short-term clinical trials have shown salmeterol to be more effective than albuterol with regular doses, as well as on demand, with similar incidence of adverse reactions. A study by Castle and associates comparing the safety of salmeterol and salbutamol in the United Kingdom noted fewer medical withdrawals due to asthma in patients taking salmeterol. This study found a small, but nonsignificant, excess mortality in the group taking salmeterol. Additional studies in patients with moderately severe asthma with inadequate symptom control despite low-to-moderate doses of inhaled steroids (eg, beclomethasone 200 mcg bid), have found greater benefit with adding salmeterol than by increasing the inhaled steroid dose (eg, beclomethasone 500 mcg bid).

A number of studies have confirmed the overall safety of daily use of salmeterol MDI and salmeterol DPI when used in addition to inhaled steroids. Studies have also shown no tolerance to the bronchodilator effects of daily salmeterol therapy for months. Experimental studies do show a decrease in the bronchoprotective effect over time; the magnitude and significance are unclear. Side effects of salmeterol may be additive with those of short-acting β-agonists. More recently, salmeterol is also available combined with fluticasone in a single DPI (Advair Diskus). The results of clinical trials of this fixed-dose combination are discussed in Chapter 11, *Add-On and Combination Therapy*.

■ Formoterol

Like salmeterol, formoterol fumarate is a long-acting, selective β_2-adrenergic agonist. It is currently available in the United States in a DPI (Foradil Aerolizer) that delivers 12 mcg of formoterol per inhalation and is approved for patients 5 and older. Like salmeterol, formoterol has 12-hour duration of action at currently approved dosages (12 mcg bid). However, formoterol differs from salmeterol in several pharmacologic properties. Formoterol has a somewhat more rapid onset of action (5 to 10 minutes) than does salmeterol (10 to 20 minutes), a difference that may be related to relative degrees of water solubility and lipophilicity that may affect diffusion to the β_2-receptor on muscle. In addition, formoterol is a full agonist whereas salmeterol is a partial agonist on the β_2-receptor.

A number of short- and long-term clinical studies have confirmed the overall efficacy and safety of daily use of formoterol when used in addition to inhaled steroids as maintenance therapy. Several studies with formoterol have found a slight attenuation of bronchodilation with continued use. After a small decrease, the level of bronchodilation was maintained. This effect appeared to be more pronounced with higher doses of formoterol (24 mcg bid vs 12 mcg bid).

Formoterol is also available combined with budesonide in a single DPI (Symbicort). The results of clinical trials with this fixed-dose combination inhaler are discussed in Chapter 11, *Add-On and Combination Therapy*.

The β-Agonist Controversy

The role of β-agonists as chronic maintenance therapy has been a subject of controversy and research for more than a decade. The concerns with chronic therapy with β-agonists include:

- Development of tolerance, as evidenced by:
  - Tachyphylaxis
  - Receptor subsensitivity
  - Diminution of peak effect
  - Reduced duration of action following repeated use
- Rebound bronchoconstriction
- Worsening asthma symptoms
- Increase in bronchial hyperreactivity.

Paradoxical bronchospasm with β-agonists has been reported rarely with both nebulizer solutions and MDIs. There were 58 reports of paradoxical bronchospasm with aerosol solutions between 1983 and 1988; and 126 reports (from 75 million canisters of β-MDIs distributed between 1985 and 1990) with β-MDIs. With aerosol solutions, benzalkonium chloride, edetate disodium, and sulfites have been implicated as a possible cause. With MDIs, emulsifying agents and preservatives, such as sorbitan, oleic acid, soy lecithin, and possibly alcohol, have been suspected. Overall, it is unlikely that the active drug or the propellants (which comprise 58% to 99% of the MDI product) play a role.

Of more import and impact on clinical practice, is the concern that chronic treatment with β-agonists may pose a risk of severe asthma episodes and possibly death. Following a July 2005 meeting of a special advisory committee, the Food and Drug Administration (FDA) issued a public health advisory alerting "health care professionals and patients that these medications may increase the chance of severe asthma episodes, and death when those episodes occur." Since this announcement, several publications, including a review by Nelson and an editorial by Martinez, have examined this issue and the potential impact of this advisory on the treatment of asthma.

Concerns regarding the use of inhaled β_2-adrenergic agonists originally arose as a result of two "epidemics" of deaths from asthma. The first arose in the United Kingdom and several other countries and lasted from 1959 through 1966. It was characterized by a 3-fold increase in deaths among patients aged 5 through 34 years. This increase in deaths was linked, at least circumstantially, to the introduction of an MDI that delivered isoproterenol at a relatively higher dose than used in other countries. Widespread publicity about the possible overuse of this drug resulted in a decrease in the death rate. Another sharp increase in asthma deaths occurred in 1976 in New Zealand. A link between the increased death rate and the use of fenoterol (a β-agonist which was prescribed at a dose relatively higher than albuterol) was suggested by several case-control studies. Again, the death rate decreased following a dramatic reduction in the use of fenoterol in New Zealand.

Subsequently, Spitzer and colleagues conducted a retrospective, matched, case-control study using a health insurance database from Saskatchewan, Canada, of a cohort of 12,301 patients for whom asthma medications had been prescribed. Data were based on matching 129 case patients who had fatal or near-fatal asthma with 655 controls. The use of β-agonists administered by an MDI was associated with an increased risk of death from asthma, with an odds ratio of 5.4 per canister of fenoterol, 2.4 per canister of albuterol, and one for background risk (ie, no fenoterol or albuterol). The primary limitation with this study (and case-control studies in general) is concern regarding the comparability of the two groups in terms of severity of underlying disease. The correlation of severity of illness with both

100

the use of inhaled β-agonists and increased mortality makes it difficult to judge the independent effect of the inhaled β-agonists from this study.

A subsequent report by the same authors, after adjusting for disease severity between the two groups, maintained that a significant correlation exists between β-agonist use and asthma mortality. No increased risk of death was associated with cromolyn sodium or ICS use.

After long-acting β-agonists were introduced outside the United States, Castle and coworkers conducted a randomized, double-blind, 16-week study in the United Kingdom that compared salmeterol with albuterol as daily therapy supplementing usual therapy in >25,000 patients. The results showed that patients who received salmeterol were three times as likely to die from asthma during the trial as those treated with albuterol (12 of 16,787 patients vs 2 of 8393 patients). This difference was not statistically significant ($P = 0.10$) since these events were so rare. Nevertheless, there was one death attributed to salmeterol for every 650 patient-years of treatment. However, interpretation of these results is not straightforward since the study was not designed to test the hypothesis that salmeterol would increase the risk of death regardless of concomitant treatment with corticosteroids. In fact, patients were randomized without consideration of their current corticosteroid therapy. In addition, there was a greater proportion of withdrawals among patients treated with albuterol, potentially introducing bias.

Given such uncertainties, the FDA requested another study to obtain additional safety data. This study, Salmeterol Multicenter Asthma Research Trial (SMART), randomized patients either to salmeterol or placebo for 28 weeks in addition to their usual therapy. Enrollment was targeted at 60,000 patients. A planned interim analysis was conducted after approximately 26,000 patients had been enrolled. At that time, although predefined criteria for stopping the study were not met, the study was terminated because of preliminary results in African American patients and difficulty in enrolling patients as a result of exclusion of any patient who had previously used a long-acting β-agonist. However, analysis of this preliminary analysis showed that asthma-related death was 4.4 times more likely in the salmeterol group as in the placebo group. Similar to the United Kingdom trial, one death was attributable to salmeterol for every 700 patient-years of treatment. Although similar numbers of patients in the two groups withdrew from the study, there are uncertainties in the interpretation of these results. Inexplicably, like the United Kingdom trial, SMART was not designed to test the hypothesis that salmeterol would increase the risk of death regardless of concomitant treatment with corticosteroids.

There have been no studies with formoterol similar to SMART. However, Mann and colleagues analyzed the results of three prospective, randomized, placebo-controlled, double-blind trials of formoterol, 12 mcg twice daily and 24 mcg twice daily. They found that more patients treated with 24 mcg of formoterol twice daily experienced more serious asthma exacerbations than did patients who received placebo. Given these findings, a 16-week, double-blind, placebo-controlled study was performed in 2085 patients with a mean forced expiratory volume in 1 second (FEV_1) of 69% of predicted value. Patients were randomized to receive 12 mcg formoterol twice daily, 24 mcg of formoterol twice daily, or 12 mcg formoterol twice daily plus up to two additional as-needed doses or placebo. The results showed that the incidence of serious adverse events was low and similar across treatment groups. However, data from all placebo-controlled trials of formoterol provided to the July 2005 FDA advisory committee by the manufacturer showed a trend toward an increased incidence of serious asthma-related events in patients who received formoterol compared with placebo.

This trend was found both among patients who used concomitant ICSs and those who did not.

In contrast to these data, a recent analysis of the trends in asthma hospitalizations and mortality in the United States from 1995 to 2002 (a period subsequent to the introduction of long-acting β-agonists) by Getahun and associates found that the rates of asthma hospitalizations and deaths decreased during this period. There is no evident explanation for this apparent discrepancy, although the increased use of ICSs as primary treatment for persistent asthma during this period may have contributed to the decrease in mortality that could have masked an increase associated with long-acting β-agonists.

Despite a substantial body of data, the β-agonist controversy is not completely resolved. Given the available evidence, it can be concluded that *regular* treatment with long-acting β-agonists is associated with increased risks of severe exacerbations and death from asthma in a small, but not inconsequential subgroup of patients.

As noted previously, the US FDA recently mandated the addition of a warning to the package inserts for all products containing LABAs referring to an increased risk of asthma-related death. It is recommended that LABAs should only be used as additional therapy for patients not adequately controlled on other asthma medications, such as low- to medium-dose corticosteroids, or whose disease severity clearly warrants initiation of treatment with two maintenance therapies, including an LABA.

Given the recent trend for the use of long-acting β-agonists in combination with ICSs, it is unfortunate that the limitations of the clinical trials performed to date do not allow any conclusions regarding the potential for ICSs to attenuate or prevent the adverse outcomes associated with the use of long-acting β-agonists. See Chapter 4, *Pathogenesis: Role of*

Airway Inflammation and Airway Reactivity for a discussion of emerging concepts in pharmacogenetics.

Theophylline

During the past decade, with the development of long-acting inhaled β-agonists and ICSs, theophylline has been relegated to a third-line drug for the management of bronchial asthma (**Table 8**.3). Theophylline has been supplanted by the other two classes of medication because it:

- Has relatively weak bronchodilating properties
- Has no clinically important anti-inflammatory properties
- Is difficult to use because of:
  - Numerous drug interactions
  - Need to monitor serum levels
  - Low therapeutic-to-toxicity ratio.

Conditions affecting blood theophylline level are listed in **Table 8**.4.

In status asthmaticus, it appears that intravenous aminophylline has little, if any, additive benefit to maximal inhaled β-agonist and corticosteroid therapy. For maintenance therapy, most patients with mild-to-moderate chronic asthma can be adequately managed with higher doses of ICSs and inhaled β-agonists. However, there are some data that show that in patients who have severe chronic asthma, chronic maintenance theophylline can have some steroid-sparing effects. Also, for a subset of patients with predominantly nocturnal asthma, a single evening dose of a long-acting theophylline preparation may be helpful. Even nocturnal asthma may be largely managed without theophylline with the aggressive use of ICSs and long-acting inhaled β-agonists.

TABLE 8.3 — Xanthine Derivatives and Combinations

Generic Name/Trade Name (Manufacturer)	Available Preparation	Suggested Dosage (Adults)
Aminophylline		
Aminophylline (many)	Injection: IV	Load: If not on theophylline at home, 5-6 mg/kg over 20 min; if on theophylline, level pending, 3 mg/kg over 20 min; a bolus of 0.5 mg/kg will increase level by 2 in the average adult. Maintenance: 0.5-0.9 mg/kg/hr
Dyphylline		
Lufyllin (many)	Tablets: 200, 400 mg; Syrup: 15 mL/100 mg	Same as theophylline below
Theophylline		
Elixophyllin (Forest)	Capsules: 100, 125, 250 mg; Elixir: 15 mL/80 mg	Normal dose range for an average adult is 300-1200 mg/day PO. Immediate-release preparations: Dose should be given q 6-8 hr. Sustained-release preparations:* Dose may be given q 12-24 hr. This dosage range is an approximate starting point; however, whenever possible, serum levels should be monitored, ie, 8 hr after a dose, after 5-6 consecutive doses. Consider the numerous conditions affecting the blood theophylline level
Theo-24 (UCB Pharma)	Capsules:* 100, 200, 300, 400 mg	
Theo-Dur (Key)	Tablets: 100, 200, 300, 450 mg; Capsules:* 50, 75 mg; Sprinkle:* 125, 200 mg	
Uniphyl (Purdue)	Tablets*: 400, 600 mg	
Abbreviations: hr, hour; IV, intravenous; min, minute; PO, orally [by mouth]; q, every.		
* Long-acting.		

8

TABLE 8.4 — Conditions Affecting Blood Theophylline Level

Decreased Clearance (increased blood level)
- Older age
- Obesity
- Chronic obstructive pulmonary disease
- Congestive heart failure
- Cirrhosis
- Acute infection, recent vaccination
- Drug interactions:
  - Allopurinol
  - Cimetidine
  - Ciprofloxacin
  - Erythromycin
  - Oral contraceptives
  - Propranolol
  - Troleandomycin
  - Zileuton

Increased Clearance (decreased blood level)
- Young age
- Active smoking
- Drug interactions:
  - Carbamazepine
  - Phenobarbital
  - Phenytoin
  - Rifampin

Anticholinergic products are shown in **Table 8.5**; however, none of these products have an FDA approval for use in treating asthma.

SUGGESTED READING

Anderson HR, Ayres JG, Sturdy PM, et al. Bronchodilator treatment and deaths from asthma: case-control study. *BMJ*. 2005;330:117.

Arkinstall WW, Atkins ME, Harrison D, Stewart JH. Once-daily sustained-release theophylline reduces diurnal variation in spirometry and symptomatology in adult asthmatics. *Am Rev Respir Dis.* 1987;135:316-321.

TABLE 8.5 — Anticholinergics*

Generic Name/Trade Name (Manufacturer)	Available Preparations	Suggested Dosage (Adults)
Ipratropium bromide		
Atrovent (Boehringer Ingelheim)	MDI: 18 mcg/puff Nebulizer solution: 0.25 mg/mL	2-4 puffs qid; Max: 12 puffs/day 0.5 mg q 4-6 hr PRN
Combivent (Boehringer Ingelheim)	MDI: 18 mcg ipratropium bromide and 103 mcg albuterol sulfate/puff	2 puffs q 6 hr
Tiotropium bromide		
Spiriva Handihaler (Pfizer/Boehringer Ingelheim)	DPI: 18 mcg/puff	1 puff daily
Abbreviations: DPI, dry-powder inhaler; FDA, Food and Drug Administration; hr, hour; MDI, metered-dose inhaler; PRN, as required; q, every; qid, four times daily.		
* These products do not have an FDA-approval for treating asthma.		

8

Backman KS, Greenberger PA, Patterson R. Airways obstruction in patients with long-term asthma consistent with "irreversible asthma." *Chest.* 1997;112:1234-1240.

Brambilla C, Le Gros V, Bourdeix I; Efficacy of Foradil in Asthma (EFORA) French Study Group. Formoterol 12 microg BID administered via single-dose dry powder inhaler in adults with asthma suboptimally controlled with salmeterol or on-demand salbutamol: a multicenter, randomized, open-label, parallel-group study. *Clin Ther.* 2003;25:2022-2036.

Buist AS, Vollmer WM. Preventing deaths from asthma. *N Engl J Med.* 1994;331:1584-1585.

Bukowskyj M, Nakatsu K, Munt PW. Theophylline reassessed. *Ann Intern Med.* 1984;101:63-73.

Castle W, Fuller R, Hall J, Palmer J. Serevent nationwide surveillance study: comparison of salmeterol with salbutamol in asthmatic patients who require regular bronchodilator treatment. *BMJ.* 1993;306:1034-1037.

Cheung D, Timmers MC, Zwinderman AH, Bel EH, Dijkman JH, Sterk PJ. Long-term effects of a long-acting beta 2-adrenoceptor agonist, salmeterol, on airway hyperresponsiveness in patients with mild asthma. *N Engl J Med.* 1992;327:1198-1203.

D'Alonzo GE, Nathan RA, Henochowicz S, Morris RJ, Ratner P, Rennard SI. Salmeterol xinafoate as maintenance therapy compared with albuterol in patients with asthma. *JAMA.* 1994;271:1412-1416.

Drazen JM, Israel E, Boushey HA, et al. Comparison of regularly scheduled with as-needed use of albuterol in mild asthma. Asthma Clinical Research Network. *N Engl J Med.* 1996;335:841-847.

Evans DJ, Taylor DA, Zetterstrom O, Chung KF, O'Connor BJ, Barnes PJ. A comparison of low-dose inhaled budesonide plus theophylline and high-dose inhaled budesonide for moderate asthma. *N Engl J Med.* 1997;337:1412-1418.

Getahun D, Demissie K, Rhoads GG. Recent trends in asthma hospitalization and mortality in the United States. *J Asthma.* 2005;42:373-378.

Grainger J, Woodman K, Pearce N, et al. Prescribed fenoterol and death from asthma in New Zealand, 1981-7: a further case-control study. *Thorax*. 1991;46:105-111.

Gray SL, Williams DM, Pulliam CC, Sirgo MA, Bishop AL, Donohue JF. Characteristics predicting incorrect metered-dose inhaler technique in older subjects. *Arch Intern Med*. 1996;156:984-988.

Greenstone IR, Ni Chroinin MN, Masse V, et al. Combination of inhaled long-acting beta2-agonists and inhaled steroids versus higher dose of inhaled steroids in children and adults with persistent asthma. *Cochrane Database Syst Rev*. 2005 Oct 19;(4):CD005533.

Lotvall J. Pharmacological similarities and differences between beta2-agonists. *Respir Med*. 2001;95(suppl B):S7-11.

Mann M, Chowdhury B, Sullivan E, Nicklas R, Anthracite R, Meyer RJ. Serious asthma exacerbations in asthmatics treated with high-dose formoterol. *Chest*. 2003;124:70-74.

Martinez FD. Safety of long-acting beta-agonists — an urgent need to clear the air. *N Engl J Med*. 2005;353:2637-2639.

Masoli M, Weatherall M, Holt S, Beasley R. Moderate dose inhaled corticosteroids plus salmeterol versus higher doses of inhaled corticosteroids in symptomatic asthma. *Thorax*. 2005;60:730-734.

McFadden ER Jr. Methylxanthines in the treatment of asthma: the rise, the fall, and the possible rise again. *Ann Intern Med*. 1991;115:323-324.

National Asthma Education and Prevention Program. Expert Panel Report: Guidelines for the Diagnosis and Management of Asthma Update on Selected Topics—2002 [published erratum appears in *J Allergy Clin Immunol*. 2003;111:466]. *J Allergy Clin Immunol*. 2002;110(suppl 5):S141-S219.

Nelson HS. Beta-adrenergic bronchodilators. *N Engl J Med*. 1995;333:499-506.

Nelson HS. Is there a problem with inhaled long-acting adrenergic agonists? *J Allergy Clin Immunol*. 2006;117:3-16.

Nelson HS, Szefler SJ, Martin RJ. Regular inhaled beta-adrenergic agonists in the treatment of bronchial asthma: beneficial or detrimental? *Am Rev Respir Dis*. 1991;144:249-250.

Nelson HS, Weiss ST, Bleecker ER, Yancey SW, Dorinsky PM; SMART Study Group. The Salmeterol Multicenter Asthma Research Trial: a comparison of usual pharmacotherapy for asthma or usual pharmacotherapy plus salmeterol. *Chest.* 2006;129:15-26.

Ni Chroinin M, Greenstone IR, Danish A, et al. Long-acting beta2-agonists versus placebo in addition to inhaled corticosteroids in children and adults with chronic asthma. *Cochrane Database Syst Rev.* 2005 Oct 19;(4):CD005535.

Pauwels RA, Lofdahl CG, Postma DS, et al. Effect of inhaled formoterol and budesonide on exacerbations of asthma. Formoterol and Corticosteroids Establishing Therapy (FACET) International Study Group. *N Engl J Med.* 1997;337:1405-1411.

Robin ED, McCauley R. Sudden cardiac death in bronchial asthma, and inhaled beta-adrenergic agonists. *Chest.* 1992;101:1699-1702.

Spitzer WO, Suissa S, Ernst P, et al. The use of beta-agonists and the risk of death and near death from asthma. *N Engl J Med.* 1992;326:501-506.

Suissa S, Ernst P, Boivin JF, et al. A cohort analysis of excess mortality in asthma and the use of inhaled beta-agonists. *Am J Respir Crit Care Med.* 1994;149:604-610.

Ulrik CS, Lange P. Decline of lung function in adults with bronchial asthma. *Am J Respir Crit Care Med.* 1994;150:629-634.

van Schayck CP, Dompeling E, van Herwaarden CL, et al. Bronchodilator treatment in moderate asthma or chronic bronchitis: continuous or on demand? A randomised controlled study. *BMJ.* 1991;303:1426-1431.

Weinberger M, Hendeles L. Theophylline in asthma. *N Engl J Med.* 1996;334:1380-1388.

Wolfe J, LaForce ST, Ziehmer B, et al. High-dose formoterol not associated with increased asthma exacerbations. *Proc Am Thorac Soc.* 2005;2:A128.

9 Anti-inflammatory Agents

Corticosteroids

Airway inflammation plays a central role in the pathogenesis of both acute and chronic asthma (see Chapter 4, *Pathogenesis: Role of Airway Inflammation and Airway Reactivity*). Therefore, anti-inflammatory agents, including corticosteroids, cromolyn sodium, and nedocromil sodium, are recommended as foundation therapy, particularly for patients with persistent symptoms. Specifically, the National Asthma Education and Prevention Program (NAEPP) guidelines (see Chapter 7, *Overview of Pharmacologic Management*), recommend inhaled corticosteroids (ICSs) as first-line therapy, followed by a stepwise addition of other agents as needed. The 2007 NAEPP guidelines reaffirm that inhaled corticosteroids are the most effective long-term control medication across all age groups. Systemic corticosteroids are reserved for the treatment of severe exacerbations and symptoms unresponsive to optimal treatment with other agents. A list of corticosteroid products currently available in the United States is shown in **Table 9**.1. When administered in significantly high doses, either inhaled or oral steroids may be equally effective. However, because therapeutically equivalent oral doses of daily or alternate-day prednisone have greater systemic side effects, ICS administration is generally preferred.

■ Mechanism of Action

Recently, new insights have been gained into the molecular mechanisms whereby corticosteroids suppress inflammation. Inflammation is characterized by the increased expression of multiple inflammatory

TABLE 9.1 — Corticosteroids

Generic Name/Trade (Manufacturer)	Available Preparations	Suggested Dosage (Adults)
Beclomethasone dipropionate		
Qvar (Teva)	MDI: 40 mcg, 80 mcg	40-60 mcg twice daily
Budesonide		
Pulmicort Turbuhaler (AstraZenaca)	DPI: 200 mcg/puff	400-1600 mcg in divided doses bid
Flunisolide		
Aerobid (Forest)	MDI: 250 mcg/puff	2 puffs bid (1 mg/day); Max: 4 puffs bid (2 mg/day)
Fluticasone propionate		
Flovent HFA (GlaxoSmithKline)	MDI: 44, 110, 220 mcg/puff	176-1760 mcg/day
Flovent Rotadisk (GlaxoSmithKline)	DPI: 50, 100, 250 mcg/puff	200-2000 mcg/day
Hydrocortisone		
Hydrocortone (Merck)	Tablets: 10 mg	20-240 mg/day

Methylprednisolone		
Medrol (Pharmacia & Upjohn)	Tablets: 4 mg	4-8 mg/day
Mometasone furoate		
Asmanex Twisthaler (Schering)	DPI: 220 mcg/puff	1 puff qd-2 puffs bid
Prednisolone		
Prelone (Muro)	Syrup: 15 mg/5 mL	5-60 mg/day
Prednisone		
Prednisone (Watson)	Tablets: 1 mg, 2.5 mg, 5 mg, 10 mg, 20 mg, 50 mg	10-50 mg/day
Triamcinolone acetonide		
Azmacort (Kos)	MDI: 100 mcg/puff	2-4 puffs bid-qid; Max: 16 puffs/day
Abbreviations: DPI, dry-powder inhaler; inh, inhalation; MDI, metered-dose inhaler.		

9

genes that are regulated by proinflammatory transcription factors that bind to and activate coactivator molecules, leading to gene transcription. Corticosteroids suppress the multiple inflammatory genes that are activated in asthmatic airways mainly by reversing activation of inflammatory genes. Activated glucocorticoid receptors also bind to recognition sites in the promoters of certain genes, resulting in secretion of anti-inflammatory proteins.

In addition, treatment with corticosteroids results in:

- Increased expression of β-adrenergic receptors on cell surfaces
- Inhibition of mediator synthesis
- Decreased cellular influx
- Stabilization of cell membranes.

Inhaled Corticosteroids

Topically active ICSs, available in the United States since the 1970s, have revolutionized the maintenance therapy for chronic asthma. These agents are administered via metered-dose inhaler (MDI) or via dry-powder inhaler (DPI). Examples of several types of MDIs and DPIs are discussed and illustrated in Chapter 12, *Inhalation Devices*. Numerous studies and wide clinical experience have shown that ICS therapy provides effective symptomatic control of chronic asthma as well as reversal of a number of parameters of airway inflammation. Both asthmatic symptoms and airflow obstruction respond to ICS therapy, usually within several weeks.

The efficacy of initial ICS therapy was demonstrated by a recent observational study by Giraud and colleagues in 396 steroid-naive patients with mild or moderate symptomatic asthma. After 4 to 8 weeks' treatment with ICSs in a dosage of 400 mcg/day to 2,000 mcg/day, achievement of asthma control, defined according to the Global Initiative for Asthma (GINA) guidelines, was assessed, and the Asthma Control Questionnaire (ACQ) was completed. The mean ICS dosage (beclomethasone equivalents) was 479 mcg/day in patients who had mild asthma (group A) and 1115 mcg/day in those with moderate asthma (group B). Asthma control was achieved in 71% of patients in group A and 65% of patients in group B. Mean ACQ score improved from 1.1 to 0.5 ($P < 0.001$) and from 2.0 to 0.8 ($P < 0.001$) in groups A and B, respectively. The authors concluded that asthma control can be achieved by ICS monotherapy for approximately two thirds of steroid-naive patients with mild-to-moderate asthma.

While ICS therapy is effective for symptomatic control, several studies have shown that it does not cure the underlying disease and, in fact, the inflammatory changes may be present even after 10 years of such therapy. Asthma symptoms frequently return with cessation of ICS therapy.

The efficacy of ICS therapy is dependent upon:
- Daily dosage
- Dosage frequency
- Delivery system
- Duration of therapy.

Over the past 5 to 10 years, the trend in the use of ICSs has been to use higher and higher doses, especially for the more severe asthmatics. This is predicated on the hypothesis that there is a dose-response effect for these agents. Although quite a number of studies support this hypothesis, there is continued debate. It is well documented that higher doses of ICSs facilitate a reduction in systemic corticosteroids in severe steroid-dependent asthma. Several studies suggest that less-frequent dosing, such as bid or qd, is effective. The less-frequent dosing has clear-cut benefits in terms of compliance. Some studies have shown a cost advantage to asthma care by the use of ICSs. Whether asthma

9

controlled by ICSs translates to decreased mortality is unknown.

Currently, there are six specific ICS products that are approved for maintenance therapy for asthma in the United States. Numerous clinical trials and expanding clinical use have shown budesonide and fluticasone to be more potent than the older agents but with comparable safety and tolerability. In addition, both of these ICSs are now available as fixed-dose, single-inhaler combinations with a long-acting β-agonist bronchodilator (see Chapter 11, *Add-On and Combination Therapy*). Most recently, mometasone furoate (Asmanex Twisthaler [DPI]) was approved by the Food and Drug Administration. Several studies have shown the efficacy and safety of mometasone 400 mcg in the evening are at least comparable to budesonide taken bid. Another once-daily agent, ciclesonide (Alvesco [HFA-MDI]), currently approved in the United Kingdom but awaiting approval in the United States has been shown to provide efficacy comparable to that of twice-daily fluticasone and budesonide.

The NAEPP Expert Panel Report Update 2002, provides a table of inhaled steroids with comparative doses to achieve a similar clinical effect (**Table 9.2**). In general, the more potent agents, such as fluticasone and budesonide, have the advantage of dosing with far fewer puffs/day to accomplish the same clinical benefit, while mometasone and ciclesonide are administered once daily. Thus the newest agents provide a significant advantage in terms of compliance.

■ Adverse Effects

The adverse effects of ICSs can be broadly classified as topical or systemic. The three main topical side effects are:

- Cough
- Oral candidiasis
- Dysphonia.

TABLE 9.2 — Estimated Comparative Daily Doses for Inhaled Corticosteroids (Adults)

Drug Name	Daily Dose (mcg)		
	Low	Medium	High
Beclomethasone HFA (40 or 80 mcg/puff)	80-240	240-480	>480
Budesonide DPI (200 mcg/inh)	200-600	600-1200	>1200
Flunisolide (250 mcg/puff)	500-1000	1000-2000	>2000
Fluticasone			
MDI: 44, 110, or 220 mcg/puff	88-264	264-660	>660
DPI: 50, 100, or 250 mcg/inh	100-300	300-600	>600
Mometasone furoate (220 mcg/puff)	220	440	880
Triamcinolone acetonide (100 mcg/puff)	400-1000	1000-2000	>2000

Abbreviations: DPI, dry-powder inhaler; inh, inhalation; MDI, metered-dose inhaler.

Modified from: National Asthma Education and Prevention Program (NAEPP) Expert Panel Report. *Guidelines for the Diagnosis and Management of Asthma—Update on Selected Topics 2002.* Bethesda, Md: US Dept of Health and Human Services; 2002. NIH publication 02-5075.

9

Slow inhalation, use of a spacer device, and mouth rinsing reduce the incidence of these side effects.

The systemic side effects may include:

- Suppression of the hypothalamic-pituitary-adrenal (HPA) axis
- Adverse effects on bone metabolism, including osteoporosis
- Slowing of growth in children and adolescents
- Bruising and dermal thinning
- Psychological changes
- Ocular hypertension and wide-angle glaucoma
- Cataract formation.

Increasingly, side effects of chronic ICS therapy are being recognized as potential problems. The factors that may contribute to toxicity include:

- Total dose
- The dosing schedule
- Whether a spacer device is used
- Whether mouth rinsing is used
- The sensitivity of the parameter used to assess systemic toxicity
- Individual susceptibility.

Studies have shown biochemical abnormalities with higher doses of ICSs. These abnormalities may be viewed as a marker for the absorption and systemic effects (toxicity) of the ICS. Parameters have included morning serum cortisol and 24-hour urinary-free cortisol excretion for HPA-axis suppression; serum osteocalcin, bone-specific serum alkaline phosphatase, urinary hydroxyproline/calcium excretion, and bone densitometry for bone metabolism (bone formation and bone resorption); and slit-lamp examination for cataract formation. The clinical significance of these subtle and sensitive markers of systemic effect, and how they translate into clinical toxicity, such as reduced bone growth, osteoporosis, or bone fractures, remain poorly established.

A variety of strategies may reduce the likelihood of systemic absorption and systemic side effects from ICSs. These include:

- Use the lowest dose that is clinically "necessary" to achieve good asthma control (eg, step down the number of puffs/day as control is achieved)
- Routinely use a spacer device with an MDI or use a DPI
- Routine mouth rinsing
- Twice-a-day dosing or dosing once a day at 4 PM or evening
- For patients requiring higher doses of ICSs, consider options for "inhaled steroid-sparing effect":
  - Long-acting β-agonists (salmeterol or formoterol)
  - Nedocromil
  - Leukotriene modifiers
  - Theophylline.

There have been rare reports of systemic eosinophilic conditions, including Churg-Strauss syndrome, in asthmatics treated with high doses of ICSs. Whether this condition is related to the ICSs or to concomitant taper of systemic steroids currently remains unknown.

Another concern with long-term ICS therapy is how it affects the decline in forced expiratory volume in 1 second (FEV_1) seen in asthma patients over time. A recent 10-year study by Lange and associates in 234 asthmatic individuals found that the decline in FEV_1 in the patients receiving ICS was 25 mL/year compared with 51 mL/year in the individuals not receiving this treatment ($P < 0.001$). A linear regression model with ICSs as the variable of interest and sex, smoking, and wheezing as covariates, showed that treatment with

ICSs was associated with a significantly ($P = 0.01$) less-steep decline in FEV_1 (18 mL/year) than without ICS treatment. Adjustment for additional variables including age, socioeconomic status, body mass index, hypersecretion of mucus, and use of other asthma medications did not change these results. Thus these results suggest that treatment with ICSs is associated with a significantly reduced, not increased, decline in ventilatory function.

■ Summary

Overall, ICSs should be considered first-line therapy for "persistent asthma" (mild, moderate, severe). However, ICSs are for chronic maintenance therapy only and not for treatment of acute asthma. The NAEPP guidelines recommend starting at a higher dose and then titrating the dose down to the minimal number of puffs to maintain chronic control (step-down therapy). We prefer more potent agents, such as fluticasone propionate, budesonide, or mometasone, for severe disease. The specific clinical roles of the newest agents, mometasone and ciclesonide, will be defined by expanding clinical experience. We routinely recommend the use of a spacer device and mouth rinsing.

Cromoglycates

■ Cromolyn Sodium

Cromolyn sodium (**Table 9.3**) is poorly absorbed orally and, therefore, is effective only when inhaled. Cromolyn sodium is available as an MDI and nebulizer solution.

Cromolyn sodium administered prior to allergen exposure blocks both the early asthmatic response (EAR) and the late-asthmatic response (LAR) following antigen inhalation. Cromolyn sodium has not demonstrated smooth muscle relaxant properties and,

TABLE 9.3 — Cromolyn Sodium/Nedocromil Sodium

Generic Name/Trade Name (Manufacturer)	Available Preparation	Suggested Dosage (Adults)
Cromolyn sodium		
Intal (King)	MDI: 800 mcg/puff	2 puffs qid
	Solution: 20 mg/2 mL ampule	1 ampule qid
Nedocromil sodium		
Tilade (King)	MDI: 1.75 mg/puff	2 puffs qid at regular intervals (14 mg/day)

Abbreviation: MDI, metered-dose inhaler; qid, four times a day.

therefore, is not a bronchodilator. It has long been held that the primary mechanism of action appears to be inhibition of mediator release from mast cells. Although the exact mechanism by which cromolyn sodium inhibits mast cell mediator release is not known, it is believed to inhibit calcium influx by phosphorylation of a membrane protein.

A large number of studies have documented the protective effect exerted by cromolyn sodium against provocative stimuli, such as:

- Allergen
- Cold air
- Sulfur dioxide
- Exercise.

The drug is most effective when administered before challenge. The protective effects against nonallergic agents such as methacholine and histamine have been less established.

Cromolyn sodium has been effective in clinical studies and in practical use for pediatric asthma, allergic asthma, and exercise-induced asthma (EIA). A number of studies have evaluated the effect of cromolyn sodium on nonspecific bronchial hyperreactivity. Studies in which cromolyn sodium was administered for >6 weeks suggest an improvement in airway reactivity. About 60% to 79% of asthmatics show a response to cromolyn sodium. A 3-month, double-blind, placebo-controlled clinical trial found that cromolyn sodium is effective for chronic adult asthma (Petty TL et al, 1989). Studies comparing cromolyn sodium and theophylline in the short-term management of chronic asthma suggest that these agents are equally effective, with perhaps greater side effects with theophylline. There are some data to show that there is an additive effect between these two agents.

A study by Shapiro and coworkers demonstrated effective symptom control with either cromolyn sodium or triamcinolone in children. However, in a 6-month trial by Toogood and colleagues involving adult asthmatics, using cromolyn sodium with beclomethasone dipropionate did not show any added clinical benefit. In contract, a recent 10-week, placebo-controlled study by Sano and associates in 251 severely asthmatic adult patients who were poorly controlled while receiving high-dose ICSs (1600 mcg/day beclomethasone equivalents) found no significant difference in morning peak expiratory flow (PEF) between patients who received the addition of nebulized cromolyn sodium (3 to 4 times/day) and those receiving placebo (saline). However, when patients were stratified into atopic and nonatopic groups, morning PEF significantly improved with cromolyn sodium in the atopic group compared with atopic controls. These results suggest that nebulized cromolyn sodium may be a useful add-on to ICSs in patients with severe atopic asthma.

9

■ Nedocromil Sodium

Nedocromil sodium is the first pyranoquinoline and is chemically distinct from all other asthma agents. A number of studies suggest that nedocromil sodium blocks both the EAR and the LAR to a variety of allergic and nonallergic asthmatic triggers. While the efficacies of nedocromil sodium and cromolyn sodium are similar in situations involving allergen exposure, nedocromil sodium is generally more potent than cromolyn sodium in protecting against nonallergic exposures. Nedocromil sodium has been shown to acutely inhibit the bronchospasm induced by several kinds of challenges, including exercise. Nedocromil sodium inhalation aerosol is not indicated for EIA in the United States. Nedocromil sodium preparation and dosing information is shown in **Table 9.3**.

Nedocromil sodium has anti-inflammatory properties on a number of cells, and *in vitro* studies suggest that nedocromil sodium may be more potent than cromolyn sodium in its cellular effects. It inhibits many cell types that are important in inflammation, including:

- Eosinophils
- Macrophages
- Mast cells
- Platelets
- Neutrophils.

There is also some suggestion that nedocromil sodium may be more potent in inhibiting bronchial C-fiber nerve endings and reducing neurogenic inflammatory mechanisms. Unlike steroids, nedocromil sodium does not get into the cell nucleus but exerts its anti-inflammatory actions at the cell surface.

A meta-analysis by Edwards and Stevens reviewed all known placebo-controlled, double-blind, randomized clinical trials involving a total of 4273 patients from 127 centers. This included both published and unpublished material. The authors compared the treatment effects of nedocromil sodium and those of placebo using efficacy variables, including:

- Symptom scores
- Peak flows
- FEV_1
- Inhaled bronchodilator use.

The numerous studies were classified by trial design into five groups. Overall, nedocromil sodium was more effective than placebo in treating asthma and of most benefit to patients receiving monotherapy with bronchodilators. The aggregate data (from meta-analysis) suggested that nedocromil sodium was less potent than ICSs. However, individual studies comparing nedocromil sodium and beclomethasone dipropionate (both given 2 puffs qid) in patients with mild-to-moderate asthma have shown comparable improvements in asthma control in this population of asthma patients (Harper GD et al, 1990; Bergmann KC

124

et al, 1989). Other studies suggest some ICS-sparing effects in patients with more severe asthma.

■ Nedocromil Sodium vs Cromolyn Sodium

Two well-controlled multicenter studies have compared the clinical efficacies of nedocromil sodium and cromolyn sodium, each administered 2 puffs qid. In a population of predominantly allergic patients who had been maintained on theophylline, the efficacies of the two drugs were similar. Statistically significant treatment differences favored cromolyn sodium for the pooled data for FEV_1 and nighttime asthma for the 5-week primary time period (Schwartz HJ et al, 1996). However, absences from work and school due to asthma, an indicator of an acute increase in asthma severity, favored nedocromil sodium over both cromolyn sodium and placebo.

In a population of predominantly nonallergic patients who had been maintained on ICSs, nedocromil sodium consistently produced greater improvements in asthma symptoms and lung function than either cromolyn sodium or placebo (Lal S et al, 1993). Statistically significant differences between the active treatments favored nedocromil sodium for daytime asthma, nighttime asthma, and nighttime bronchodilator use. These findings are perhaps not surprising in light of the results of clinical pharmacologic comparisons of the two drugs; however, currently available data on the relative efficacy of the two drugs are inconclusive.

Anti-inflammatory Therapy: Summary

Overall, inflammatory agents, particularly ICSs, should be the foundation of maintenance therapy for most patients with chronic asthma. For mild-to-moderate asthma, low-to-moderate doses of ICSs, leukotriene modifiers, cromolyn sodium, and nedocromil sodium are effective. In patients where there is concern for toxicity of ICSs (eg, in patients requiring high doses of ICSs, in children, and in postmenopausal women), cromolyn sodium, nedocromil sodium, or antileukotrienes represent a rational alternative. Also, for patients who continue to be symptomatic despite moderate doses of ICSs, the current guidelines recommend the addition of a long-acting β-agonist bronchodilator (salmeterol, formoterol), or alternately:

- Leukotriene modifiers
- Cromolyn sodium
- Nedocromil sodium
- Methylxanthines

SUGGESTED READING

Cromolyn Sodium/Nedocromil Sodium

Bergmann KC, Bauer CP, Overlack A. A placebo-controlled, blind comparison of nedocromil sodium and beclomethasone dipropionate in bronchial asthma. *Curr Med Res Opin.* 1989;11:533-542.

Callaghan B, Teo NC, Clancy L. Effects of the addition of nedocromil sodium to maintenance bronchodilator therapy in the management of chronic asthma. *Chest.* 1992;101:787-792.

Edwards AM, Stevens MT. The clinical efficacy of inhaled nedocromil sodium (Tilade) in the treatment of asthma. *Eur Respir J.* 1993;6:35-41.

Harper GD, Neill P, Vathenen AS, Cookson JB, Ebden P. A comparison of inhaled beclomethasone dipropionate and nedocromil sodium as additional therapy in asthma. *Respir Med.* 1990;84:463-469.

Hoag JE, McFadden ER Jr. Long-term effect of cromolyn sodium on nonspecific bronchial hyperresponsiveness: a review. *Ann Allergy.* 1991;66:53-63.

Kuzemko JA. Twenty years of sodium cromoglycate treatment: a short review. *Respir Med.* 1989;83(suppl A):11-14.

Lal S, Dorow PD, Venho KK, Chatterjee SS. Nedocromil sodium is more effective than cromolyn sodium for the treatment of chronic reversible obstructive airway disease. *Chest.* 1993;104:438-447.

McFadden ER Jr, Gilbert IA. Exercise-induced asthma. *N Engl J Med*. 1994;330:1362-1367.

Murphy S, Kelly HW. Cromolyn sodium: a review of mechanisms and clinical use in asthma. *Drug Intell Clin Pharm*. 1987;21:22-35.

North American Tilade Study Group. A double-blind multicenter group comparative study of the efficacy and safety of nedocromil sodium in the management of asthma. *Chest*. 1990;97:1299-1306.

Petty TL, Rollins DR, Christopher K, Good JT, Oakley R. Cromolyn sodium is effective in adult Chronic asthmatics. *Am Rev Respir Dis*. 1989;139:694-701.

Sano Y, Adachi M, Kiuchi T, Miyamoto T. Effects of nebulized sodium cromoglycate on adult patients with severe refractory asthma. *Respir Med*. 2006;100:420-433.

Schwartz HJ, Blumenthal M, Brady R, et al. A comparative study of the clinical efficacy of nedocromil sodium and placebo. How does cromolyn sodium compare as an active control treatment? *Chest*. 1996;109:945-952.

Shapiro GG, Sharpe M, DeRouen TA, et al. Cromolyn versus triamcinolone acetonide for youngsters with moderate asthma. *J Allergy Clin Immunol*. 1991;88:742-748.

Toogood JH, Jennings B, Lefcoe NM. A clinical trial of combined cromolyn/beclomethasone treatment for chronic asthma. *J Allergy Clin Immunol*. 1981;67:317-324.

Inhaled Corticosteroids

Barnes PJ. Corticosteroids: The drugs to beat. *Eur J Pharmacol*. 2006;533:2-14.

Barnes PJ, Pedersen S, Busse WW. Efficacy and safety of inhaled corticosteroids. New developments. *Am J Respir Crit Care Med*. 1998;157(suppl):S1-S53.

Boorsma M, Andersson N, Larsson P, Ullman A. Assessment of the relative systemic potency of inhaled fluticasone and budesonide. *Eur Respir J*. 1996;9:1427-1432.

Boulet LP, Drollmann A, Magyar P, et al. Comparative efficacy of once-daily ciclesonide and budesonide in the treatment of persistent asthma. *Respir Med*. 2006;100(5):785-794.

Buhl R, Vinkler I, Magyar P, et al. Comparable efficacy of ciclesonide once daily versus fluticasone propionate twice daily in asthma. *Pulm Pharmacol Ther*. 2006;19(6):404-412.

Cumming RG, Mitchell P, Leeder SR. Use of inhaled corticosteroids and the risk of cataracts. *N Engl J Med*. 1997;337:8-14.

D'Urzo A, Karpel JP, Busse WW, et al. Efficacy and safety of mometasone furoate administered once-daily in the evening in patients with persistent asthma dependent on inhaled corticosteroids. *Curr Med Res Opin*. 2005;21:1281-1289.

Gibson PG, Powell H. Initial corticosteroid therapy for asthma. *Curr Opin Pulm Med*. 2006;12:48-53.

Hubner M, Hochhaus G, Derendorf H. Comparative pharmacology, bioavailability, pharmacokinetics, and pharmacodynamics of inhaled glucocorticosteroids. *Immunol Allergy Clin North Am*. 2005;25:469-88.

Johnson M. Pharmacodynamics and pharmacokinetics of inhaled glucocorticoids. *J Allergy Clin Immunol*. 1996;97:169-176.

Juniper EF, Kline PA, Vanzieleghem MA, Ramsdale EH, O'Byrne PM, Hargreave FE. Effect of long-term treatment with an inhaled corticosteroid (budesonide) on airway hyperresponsiveness and clinical asthma in nonsteroid-dependent asthmatics. *Am Rev Respir Dis*. 1990;142:832-836.

Kamada AK, Szefler SJ, Martin RJ, et al. Issues in the use of inhaled glucocorticoids. The Asthma Clinical Research Network. *Am J Respir Crit Care Med*. 1996;153:1739-1748.

Karpel JP, Busse WW, Noonan MJ, Monahan ME, Lutsky B, Staudinger H. Effects of mometasone furoate given once daily in the evening on lung function and symptom control in persistent asthma. *Ann Pharmacother*. 2005;39:1977-1983.

Lange P, Scharling H, Ulrik CS, Vestbo J. Inhaled corticosteroids and decline of lung function in community residents with asthma. *Thorax*. 2006;61:100-104.

Li JT, Reed CE. Proper use of aerosol corticosteroids to control asthma. *Mayo Clin Proc*. 1989;64:205-210.

National Asthma Education and Prevention Program. Expert Panel Report: Guidelines for the Diagnosis and Management of Asthma Update on Selected Topics—2002 [published erratum appears in *J Allergy Clin Immunol*. 2003;111:466]. *J Allergy Clin Immunol*. 2002;110(suppl 5):S141-S219.

Niphadkar P, Jagannath K, Joshi JM, et al. Comparison of the efficacy of ciclesonide 160 microg QD and budesonide 200 microg BID in adults with persistent asthma: a phase III, randomized, double-dummy, open-label study. *Clin Ther*. 2005;27:1752-1763.

Noonan M, Chervinsky P, Busse WW, et al. Fluticasone propionate reduces oral prednisone use while it improves asthma control and quality of life. *Am J Respir Crit Care Med*. 1995;152:1467-1473.

Pearlman DS, Berger WE, Kerwin E, Laforce C, Kundu S, Banerji D. Once-daily ciclesonide improves lung function and is well tolerated by patients with mild-to-moderate persistent asthma. *J Allergy Clin Immunol*. 2005;116:1206-1212.

Selroos O, Pietinalho A, Lofroos AB, Riska H. Effect of early vs late intervention with inhaled corticosteroids in asthma. *Chest*. 1995;108:1228-1234.

Tattersfield AE, Harrison TW, Hubbard RB, Mortimer K. Safety of inhaled corticosteroids. *Proc Am Thorac Soc*. 2004;1:171-175.

Toogood JH. Complications of topical steroid therapy for asthma. *Am Rev Respir Dis*. 1990;141(suppl):S89-S96.

Wardlaw A, Larivee P, Eller J, Cockcroft DW, Ghaly L, Harris AG. Efficacy and safety of mometasone furoate dry powder inhaler vs fluticasone propionate metered-dose inhaler in asthma subjects previously using fluticasone propionate. *Ann Allergy Asthma Immunol*. 2004;93:49-55.

Woolcock A, Lundback B, Ringdal N, Jacques LA. Comparison of addition of salmeterol to inhaled steroids with doubling of the dose of inhaled steroids. *Am J Respir Crit Care Med*. 1996;153:1481-1488.

9

10
Leukotriene Modifiers

The cysteinyl leukotrienes (LTC_4, LTD_4, and LTE_4), formally known as the slow-reacting substance of anaphylaxis, are formed by the lipoxygenation of arachidonic acid by the enzyme 5-lipoxygenase (**Figure 10.1**). These compounds, released by mast cells, eosinophils, and airway epithelial cells, have a variety of potent effects, including:

- Bronchoconstriction
- Increased permeability
- Enhanced airway reactivity.

Considerable evidence accumulated over nearly 2 decades suggest that the cysteinyl leukotrienes are involved in the pathogenesis of experimentally induced asthma as well as spontaneously occurring chronic human asthma. Leukotrienes can be recovered from:

- Nasal secretions
- Bronchoalveolar lavage fluid
- Urine of patients with asthma.

A number of potent agents, including competitive receptor antagonists and those that interfere with leukotriene synthesis, have been and continue to be developed. These agents inhibit asthmatic responses to:

- Allergens
- Exercise
- Cold, dry air
- Aspirin.

Three agents that antagonize leukotriene binding or interfere with its synthesis were approved in the United States in 1997 and 1998 for use as maintenance therapy for asthma (**Table 10.1**). A fourth agent, pran-

FIGURE 10.1 — Leukotriene Pathway

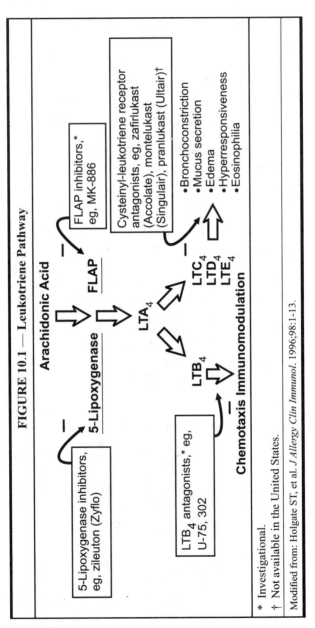

* Investigational.
† Not available in the United States.

Modified from: Holgate ST, et al. *J Allergy Clin Immunol.* 1996;98:1-13.

TABLE 10.1 — Comparison of Antileukotrienes

Considerations	Zafirlukast (Accolate)	Zileuton (Zyflo)	Montelukast (Singulair)
Age	≥12 years	≥12 years	≥6 years
Usual dose	20 mg bid	600 mg qid	10 mg qd in the evening (adults); 5-mg chewable tablets (children)
Mechanism	Blocks the LTD_4 receptor	Inhibits 5-lipoxygenase	Blocks the cys-LT_1 or LTD_4 receptor
Warnings	? CSS ? LFTs	Increased LFTs, monitor LFTs 7 times in first year	? CSS
Metabolism	P-450: 3A4, 2C9	P-450: 1A2, 3A4, 2C9	P-450: 3A4, 2C9
Dosing considerations	Empty stomach (1 hour before or 2 hours after); food decreases absorption by 40%	None	None
Drug interactions	Warfarin (↑ PT) Phenytoin, carbamazepine	Warfarin (↑ PT) Theophylline (↑) Propranolol (↑)	None

Abbreviations: bid, twice a day; CSS, Churg-Strauss syndrome; cys-LT1, cysteinyl leukotriene; LFT, liver function test; LTD_4, leukotriene D_4; P-450, cytochrome enzyme; PT, prothrombin time; qd, every day; qid, four times a day.

lukast, has been approved in Japan, and several others are in various stages of development.

Controlled clinical trials with the currently used leukotriene modifiers have demonstrated their efficacy in improving pulmonary function, reducing symptoms, decreasing nighttime awakenings, and decreasing the need for rescue medications. They exert anti-inflammatory effects that attenuate cellular infiltration and bronchial hyperresponsiveness and complement the anti-inflammatory properties of inhaled corticosteroids. In patients with exercise-induced asthma, leukotriene modifiers limit the decline in and quicken the recovery of pulmonary function without the tolerance issues seen with chronic long-acting β-adrenoceptor agonist use. In patients with aspirin (acetylsalicylic acid)-induced asthma, they improve pulmonary function and shift the dose-response curve to the right, reducing the patient's response to aspirin. These agents are generally safe and well tolerated with adverse effect profiles similar to that of placebo.

Montelukast

Montelukast (Singulair) is a potent and specific cysteinyl leukotriene (cys-LT_1 or LTD_4) receptor antagonist. Montelukast may have several advantages compared with zafirlukast or zileuton (**Table 10.1**). These include ease of dosing (once a day; no significant change in absorption by food) and absence of significant drug interactions. Clinical experience to date shows an excellent safety profile with no effect on liver function tests. As with zafirlukast, postmarketing surveillance has identified several case reports of eosinophilic conditions, including Churg-Strauss syndrome. Whether this condition is related to montelukast or to a concomitant taper of systemic steroids remains unknown. Also, the 5-mg chewable tablets have been used in 6- to 14-year-old asthmatics with efficacy and safety.

Several published studies indicate that montelukast 10 mg given once daily at bedtime causes significant improvement in chronic mild-to-moderate asthma compared with placebo. A 3-month, double-blind, parallel-group study (n=681 with forced expiratory volume in 1 second [FEV_1] 50% to 80%) showed significant improvement in the montelukast group (asthma exacerbation decreased by 31%, asthma-free days increased by 37%). Another randomized trial involving adults with moderate-to-severe asthma (n=226) showed that montelukast 10 mg allowed significant tapering of inhaled steroids in patients requiring moderate-to-high doses. A 4-week, controlled trial in 80 aspirin-intolerant adult asthmatics showed that montelukast 10 mg given at bedtime significantly improved asthma control.

Finally, an 8-week, randomized, double-blind study was completed in children (age 6 to 14 years) with mild-to-moderate asthma (FEV_1 50% to 80%). Mean FEV_1 increased from 1.85 L to 2.01 L (8.23%) in the montelukast group and 1.85 L to 1.93 L (3.58%) in the placebo group (P <0.001). Secondary parameters (ie, as-needed β-agonist use and percentage of days and patients with an exacerbation) also improved significantly in the montelukast group.

Variability in clinical response to montelukast among individual patients has been reported. A recent study by Lima and colleagues examined the influence of leukotriene-pathway polymorphisms on response to montelukast in patients with asthma who received montelukast for 6 months in a clinical trial. Among several polymorphisms, associations were found between genotypes of single nucleotide polymorphisms (SNPs) in two genes and changes in FEV_1 (P <0.05), and between two SNPs in two other genes and exacerbation rates. Associations between several haplotypes and risk of exacerbations were also found. Therefore, genetic variation in leukotriene-pathway candidate genes contributes to variability in montelukast response.

10

Zafirlukast

Zafirlukast (Accolate) is a selective, competitive receptor antagonist at the LTD_4 and LTE_4 level. Three US, double-blind, randomized, placebo-controlled, 13-week studies in 1380 patients with mild-to-moderate asthma showed that treatment with zafirlukast improved:

- Daytime asthma symptoms
- Nighttime awakenings
- Morning asthma symptoms
- Rescue albuterol use
- FEV_1
- Morning peak expiratory flow rate.

A 6-week, double-blind, controlled trial of moderate asthma (FEV_1 40% to 75% prior to therapy with β-agonist alone or with theophylline) involved 67 patients treated with 20 mg zafirlukast bid. Compared with baseline measurements, zafirlukast:

- Decreased night awakenings by 46%
- Decreased albuterol use by 30%
- Decreased daytime symptoms by 26%
- Increased FEV_1 by 11%.

A 13-week, controlled trial of mild-to-moderate asthmatics compared the effectiveness of zafirlukast 20 mg bid (n=103) vs placebo (n=43) when added to as-needed short-acting β-agonist. Zafirlukast therapy was more effective by a variety of clinical and economic parameters:

- 89% more days without symptoms (7.0 vs 3.7 days/month, $P = 0.03$)
- 89% more days without use of β-agonists (11.3 vs 6.0 days/month, $P = 0.001$)
- 55% fewer health care contacts (18.5 vs 40.7 per 100/month, $P = 0.007$)

- 55% fewer days of absence from work or school (15.6 vs 35 per 100/month, $P = 0.04$).

Presumably these results were noted even without a significant improvement in FEV_1.

Zafirlukast is administered as 20 mg bid and is well absorbed orally. It should be given on an empty stomach; otherwise, drug levels may be reduced by 40%. At the currently recommended dose, the risk of liver function abnormalities appears to be quite low and routine monitoring is unnecessary. However, there have been isolated reports of liver function abnormalities. These abnormalities become more prominent at higher doses (eg, 80 mg/day). Also, a recent study described eight patients with Churg-Strauss vasculitis syndrome after starting zafirlukast for oral steroid-dependent asthma. All but one of these patients were on systemic corticosteroids and this syndrome occurred with tapering or discontinuation of steroid therapy. Whether this complication is related to zafirlukast or to tapering of systemic steroids is unknown.

Zileuton

Zileuton (Zyflo) is a synthesis inhibitor that blocks the 5-lipoxygenase enzyme, thus interfering with production of the cysteinyl leukotrienes as well as LTB_4. Zileuton is approved for use as a 600 mg tablet qid. This medication can be taken with food. Studies suggest that there is a 5% incidence of liver function abnormalities. It is recommended that baseline alanine aminotransferase (ALT) be measured as well as follow-up monitoring approximately seven times during the first year. Many patients with liver function abnormalities may continue to take the drug. Several placebo-controlled, clinical trials show significant benefit with the use of this agent.

137

A 4-week trial was conducted in 139 asthmatics (FEV$_1$ 40% to 70%) not on inhaled or oral steroids. Patients were randomized to zileuton 2.4 g/day, 1.6 g/day, or placebo. Zileuton produced a 14.6% increase in FEV$_1$ within 1 hour of administration (P <0.001) compared with placebo and a 13.4% increase after 4 weeks (P = 0.02). Improvement was greater at the higher dose. A 13-week study included 401 patients with mild-to-moderate asthma randomized to 600 mg, 400 mg, or placebo qid. Patients on 600 mg experienced significantly fewer exacerbations requiring oral steroids (6.1% vs 15.6%, P = 0.02), suggesting anti-inflammatory action. Average FEV$_1$ improved 15.7% in the 600-mg group vs 7.7% in the placebo group (P = 0.006).

Clinical Role for Leukotriene Modifiers

Table 10.2 shows a comparison of the clinical properties of inhaled corticosteroids (ICSs) leukotriene modifiers. While leukotriene modifiers provide some advantages, the 2007 National Asthma Education and Prevention Program (NAEPP) guidelines recommend ICSs as the preferred first-line therapy for all patients with persistent asthma. However, leukotriene modifiers are recommended as an alternate initial therapy in patients with mild persistent asthma (see Chapter 7, *Overview of Pharmacologic Management*).

A recent systematic review of the clinical literature assessed the efficacy and safety of leukotriene modifiers as first-line therapy vs an ICS. Ng and associates analyzed the results of 27 trials in patients with mild-to-moderate persistent asthma who received either an ICS or a leukotriene modifier as initial therapy. In most trials, daily dose of ICS was 400 mcg beclomethasone or equivalent. Patients treated with leukotriene modifiers were 65% more likely to experience an exacerbation requiring systemic steroids (relative risk 1.65).

TABLE 10.2 — Comparison of the Clinical Properties of Inhaled Steroids and Antileukotrienes

Criteria	Inhaled Steroids	Antileukotrienes
Available since	1970s	1997-1998
Logistics of patient use with compliance	Complex (proper MDI technique, spacers, multiple MDIs)	Simple (qd pill)
Magnitude of acute/subacute response	None	Moderate (onset 1-2 hours; 5% to 10% increase in FEV_1)
Magnitude of chronic response	15% to 25% increase in FEV_1	10% to 14% increase in FEV_1
Effect on airway hyper-responsiveness	Moderate (2-3 doubling doses)*	Unknown
Anti-inflammatory effect	Nonspecific; well established	Very specific; limited data
Safety	Both topical and systemic steroid side effects; dependent on dose, duration, use of spacer/mouth rinsing, susceptibility, etc; CSS (fluticasone)	Generally safe; LFT elevations (zileuton) and CSS (zafirlukast, montelukast); see text for details
Oral steroid-sparing effect	Definite	Probable (zileuton)

Abbreviations: CSS, Churg-Strauss syndrome; FEV_1, forced expiratory volume in 1 second; LFT, liver function tests; MDI, metered-dose inhaler; qd, once per day.

* Nonspecific airway hyperresponsiveness as assessed by methacholine or histamine bronchoprovocation.

10

Significant differences favoring an ICS were noted in secondary outcomes, including improvements in FEV_1, symptoms, nocturnal awakenings, rescue medication use, symptom-free days, and quality of life. In addition, leukotriene-modifier therapy was associated with 160% increased risk of withdrawals due to poor asthma control. This review did not identify any difference in short-term safety between ICSs and leukotriene modifiers. However, adverse effects typically associated with an ICS (such as growth suppression, osteopenia, and adrenal suppression) were not measured, preventing a fair comparison of the safety profile on long-term use. Therefore, the scientific evidence so far does not support the substitution of leukotriene modifiers for low doses of an ICS.

The EPR–Update 2002 also recommends leukotriene modifiers as an alternative to a long-acting β-agonist (LABA) as an adjunct to ICSs in patients with moderate or severe asthma. As discussed in more detail in Chapter 11, *Add-On and Combination Therapy*, several studies and meta-analyses have shown that adjunctive LABAs (currently salmeterol or formoterol) are more effective than leukotriene modifiers.

In summary, it is likely that ICSs have more potent effects, especially in patients with moderate-to-severe disease. However, a major cause for poor asthma outcome is patient noncompliance with prescribed inhaled steroid therapy. Once- or twice-a-day oral therapy with the leukotriene modifiers offers a significant compliance advantage. Montelukast represents a significant advance for pediatric asthmatics, being approved as a 5-mg chewable tablet for use once a day in ages 6 to 14. The antileukotrienes may facilitate a reduction in the need for inhaled β-agonists and ICSs, thereby minimizing well-known side effects. Similar to what is seen with other classes of asthma medications (including ICSs), there is a subset of patients who respond much more dramatically to the leukotriene modifiers, usually within the first 30 days. If there is no response within 1 to 3 months, it is reasonable to stop these agents. Furthermore, leukotriene modifiers may be particularly beneficial as the drug of choice in a small subset of patients with aspirin-sensitive asthma. They may also have a secondary benefit in patients with exercise-induced asthma, where leukotrienes are important mediators of disease.

SUGGESTED READING

Ceylan E, Gencer M, Aksoy S. Addition of formoterol or montelukast to low-dose budesonide: an efficacy comparison in short- and long-term asthma control. *Respiration.* 2004;71:594-601.

Creticos PS. Treatment options for initial maintenance therapy of persistent asthma: a review of inhaled corticosteroids and leukotriene receptor antagonists. *Drugs.* 2003;63(suppl 2):1-20.

Dahlen B, Nizankowska E, Szczeklik A, et al. Benefits from adding the 5-lipoxygenase inhibitor zileuton to conventional therapy in aspirin-intolerant asthmatics. *Am J Respir Crit Care Med.* 1998;157:1187-1194.

Ducharme F, Hicks G, Kakuma R. Addition of anti-leukotriene agents to inhaled corticosteroids for chronic asthma. *Cochrane Database Syst Rev.* 2002;(1):CD003133. Update in: *Cochrane Database Syst Rev.* 2004;(2):CD003133.

Ducharme FM. Inhaled corticosteroids versus leukotriene antagonists as first-line therapy for asthma: a systematic review of current evidence. *Treat Respir Med.* 2004;3:399-405.

Ducharme FM, Hicks GC. Anti-leukotriene agents compared to inhaled corticosteroids in the management of recurrent and/or chronic asthma in adults and children. *Cochrane Database Syst Rev.* 2002;(3):CD002314. Update in: *Cochrane Database Syst Rev.* 2004;(2):CD002314.

Holgate ST, Bradding P, Sampson AP. Leukotriene antagonists and synthesis inhibitors: new directions in asthma therapy. *J Allergy Clin Immunol.* 1996;98:1-13.

10

Ilowite J, Webb R, Friedman B, et al. Addition of montelukast or salmeterol to fluticasone for protection against asthma attacks: a randomized, double-blind, multicenter study. *Ann Allergy Asthma Immunol.* 2004;92:641-648.

Israel E, Cohn J, Dube L, Drazen JM. Effect of treatment with zileuton, a 5-lipoxygenase inhibitor, in patients with asthma. A randomized controlled trial. Zileuton Clinical Trial Group. *JAMA.* 1996;275:931-936.

Israel E, Rubin P, Kemp JP, et al. The effect of inhibition of 5-lipoxygenase by zileuton in mild-to-moderate asthma. *Ann Intern Med.* 1993;119:1059-1066.

Kavuru MS, Subramony R, Vann AR. Antileukotrienes and asthma: alternative or adjunct to inhaled steroids? *Cleve Clin J Med.* 1998;65:519-526.

Kemp JP. Recent advances in the management of asthma using leukotriene modifiers. *Am J Respir Med.* 2003;2:139-156.

Knorr B, Matz J, Bernstein JA, et al. Montelukast for chronic asthma in 6- to 14-year-old children: a randomized, double-blind trial. Pediatric Montelukast Study Group. *JAMA.* 1998;279:1181-1186.

Lakomski PG, Chitre M. Evaluation of the utilization patterns of leukotriene modifiers in a large managed care health plan. *J Manag Care Pharm.* 2004;10:115-121.

Leff JA, Busse WW, Pearlman D, et al. Montelukast, a leukotriene-receptor antagonist, for the treatment of mild asthma and exercise-induced bronchoconstriction. *N Engl J Med.* 1998;339:147-152.

Leff JA, Israel E, Noonan MJ, et al. Montelukast allows tapering of inhaled corticosteroids in asthmatic patients while maintaining clinical stability. *Am J Respir Crit Care Med.* 1997;155:A976.

Lima JJ, Zhang S, Grant A, et al. Influence of leukotriene pathway polymorphisms on response to montelukast in asthma. *Am J Respir Crit Care Med.* 2006;173:379-385.

Malmstrom K, Rodriguez-Gomez G, Guerra J, et al. Oral montelukast, inhaled beclomethasone, and placebo for chronic asthma. A randomized, controlled trial. Montelukast/Beclomethasone Study Group. *Ann Intern Med.* 1999;130:487-495.

Meltzer SS, Hasday JD, Cohn J, Bleecker ER. Inhibition of exercise-induced bronchospasm by zileuton: a 5-lipoxygenase inhibitor. *Am J Respir Crit Care Med.* 1996;153:931-935.

National Asthma Education and Prevention Program. Expert Panel Report: Guidelines for the Diagnosis and Management of Asthma Update on Selected Topics—2002 [published erratum appears in *J Allergy Clin Immunol.* 2003;111;466]. *J Allergy Clin Immunol.* 2002;(suppl 5):S141-S219.

Noonan MJ, Chervinsky P, Brandon M, et al. Montelukast, a potent leukotriene receptor antagonist, causes dose-related improvements in chronic asthma. Montelukast Asthma Study Group. *Eur Respir J.* 1998;11:1232-1239.

O'Byrne PM, Israel E, Drazen JM. Antileukotrienes in the treatment of asthma. *Ann Intern Med.* 1997;127:472-480.

Reiss TF, Altman LC, Chervinsky P, et al. Effects of montelukast (MK-0476), a new potent cysteinyl leukotriene (LTD4) receptor antagonist, in patients with chronic asthma. *J Allergy Clin Immunol.* 1996;98:528-534.

Reiss TF, Chervinsky P, Dockhorn RJ, Shingo S, Seidenberg B, Edwards TB. Montelukast, a once-daily leukotriene receptor antagonist, in the treatment of chronic asthma: a multicenter, randomized, double-blind trial. Montelukast Clinical Research Study Group. *Arch Intern Med.* 1998;158:1213-1220.

Reiss TF, Sorkness CA, Stricker W, et al. Effects of montelukast (MK-0476); a potent cysteinyl leukotriene receptor antagonist, on bronchodilation in asthmatic subjects treated with and without inhaled corticosteroids. *Thorax.* 1997;52:45-48.

Riccioni G, Della Vecchia R, Di Ilio C, D'Orazio N. Effect of the two different leukotriene receptor antagonists, montelukast and zafirlukast, on quality of life: a 12-week randomized study. *Allergy Asthma Proc.* 2004;25:445-448.

Schwartz HJ, Petty T, Dube LM, Swanson LJ, Lancaster JF. A randomized controlled trial comparing zileuton with theophylline in moderate asthma. The Zileuton Study Group. *Arch Intern Med.* 1998;158:141-148.

Suissa S, Dennis R, Ernst P, Sheehy O, Wood-Dauphinee S. Effectiveness of the leukotriene receptor antagonist zafirlukast for mild-to-moderate asthma. A randomized, double-blind, placebo-controlled trial. *Ann Intern Med.* 1997;126:177-183.

Wechsler ME, Garpestad E, Flier SR, et al. Pulmonary infiltrates, eosinophilia, and cardiomyopathy following corticosteroid withdrawal in patients with asthma receiving zafirlukast. *JAMA.* 1998;279:455-457.

11 Add-On and Combination Therapy

The current National Asthma Education and Prevention Program (NAEPP) evidence-based guidelines recommend a stepwise approach to pharmacologic management of patients with persistent asthma (see Chapter 7, *Overview of Pharmacologic Management*). In this approach, a daily low dose of an inhaled corticosteroid (ICS) is the preferred, first-line therapy for patients with mild, persistent asthma, followed by increases in ICS dose and/or the addition of one or more other agent as needed according to the severity of the disease. Thus many patients, particularly those with persistent moderate-to-severe asthma, require two or more separate medications in addition to the occasional use of short-acting β-agonist rescue agents, a situation that can complicate adherence. Two preparations containing an ICS and a long-acting β-agonist (LABA) in a single inhaler are available in the United States (Advair and Symbicort). The clinical trial experience with various combination regimens is reviewed below.

Inhaled Corticosteroids and Long-Acting β-Agonists

The combination of an ICS and an LABA is increasingly used as maintenance therapy in patients with persistent moderate-to-severe asthma. The main effect of ICSs is thought to be mediated through suppression of airway inflammation, while LABAs are thought to work by inducing bronchodilation.

However, there are emerging data to indicate that these two classes of drugs may interact positively with each other, leading to added or perhaps synergistic benefits for patients. Corticosteroids enhance the expression of β_2-adrenoceptors, thus providing protection against desensitization and development of tolerance to LABAs, which may occur with prolonged use of these medications. LABAs, on the other hand, may amplify the anti-inflammatory effects of corticosteroids by accelerating nuclear translocation of the glucocorticoid receptor complex, and enhancing transcription and expression of steroid-inducible genes in proinflammatory cells.

■ Add-On Administration

The stepwise approach begins with a daily low dose of ICS. However, when this regimen does not provide adequate symptom control, a decision must be made whether to increase the ICS dose or add a second medication, typically an LABA. Several recent systematic reviews have examined the clinical trial evidence regarding the following clinical questions: (1) addition of LABA vs placebo; (2) addition of LABA vs increase in ICS dose; (3) does the addition of LABA have an ICS-sparing effect; and (4) ICS/LABA combination vs ICS as first-line therapy.

Addition of LABA vs Placebo

Ni and associates analyzed the results of 26 randomized, controlled clinical trials that compared the addition of an inhaled LABA (formoterol or salmeterol) to ICS (200 to 400 mcg/day beclomethasone or equivalent) with an ICS alone for asthma therapy in children aged 2 years and above (eight trials) and in adults (18 trials). The primary end point was the rate of asthma exacerbations requiring systemic corticosteroids. Secondary end points included pulmonary function tests, symptom scores, adverse events, and withdrawal rates. The results of this analysis showed that the addition of a daily LABA reduced the risk of exacerbations requiring systemic steroids by 19% (relative risk [RR] 0.81). The addition of an LABA also significantly improved forced expiratory volume in 1 second (FEV_1) (weighted mean difference 170 mL) and increased the proportion of symptom-free days by 17% and rescue-free days by 19%. The group treated with an LABA plus an ICS showed a reduction in the use of rescue short-acting β-agonists and experienced fewer withdrawals due to poor asthma control. There was no group difference in risk of overall adverse effects (RR 0.98), withdrawals due to adverse events, or specific adverse events.

Addition of LABA vs Increase in ICS Dose

Greenstone and associates reviewed 30 (three pediatric, 27 adult) randomized, controlled, clinical trials that compared the addition of an LABA with an increased ICS dose in trials that enrolled 9509 patients who were symptomatic, generally presenting with moderate (FEV_1 60% to 79% of predicted) airway obstruction. These trials assessed the addition of salmeterol (22 trials) or formoterol (eight trials) with a median of 400 mcg beclomethasone or equivalent ICS compared with a median of 800 to 1000 mcg/day beclomethasone-equivalent ICS. There was no significant group difference in the rate of patients with exacerbations requiring systemic corticosteroids. The combination of an LABA and an ICS resulted in greater improvement from baseline in FEV_1, in symptom-free days, and in the daytime use of rescue β- agonists than the higher dose of ICS alone. With the exception of a 3-fold increased rate of tremor in the LABA group, there was no significant group difference in the rate of overall adverse events or specific side effects. The rate of withdrawals due to poor asthma control favored the combination of an LABA and an ICS. Overall, combination therapy resulted in greater improvement in lung function, symptoms, and use of rescue medications.

Another recent meta-analysis by Masoli and colleagues analyzed the results of 12 randomized, double-blind clinical trials that compared the efficacy of adding salmeterol to moderate doses of an ICS (fluticasone propionate 200 mcg/day or equivalent) with increasing the ICS dose by at least 2-fold in 4576 symptomatic adult patients with asthma. The main outcome measures were the number of subjects withdrawn from the study due to asthma and the number of subjects with at least one moderate or severe exacerbation. The number of subjects withdrawn due to asthma and with at least one moderate or severe exacerbation was higher in the high-dose ICS group. For the secondary outcome variables (FEV_1 morning and evening peak expiratory flow (PEF), and daytime rescue β-agonist use) there was significantly greater benefit in the salmeterol combination group.

Does the Addition of an LABA Have an ICS-Sparing Effect?

Gibson and coworkers sought to determine if adding an LABA to a moderate-to-high dose of an ICS would result in a reduction of maintenance ICS dose without loss of asthma control. A total of 19 publications describing 10 trials in adult asthmatics were included in this review. Studies that compared a reduced-dose (mean 60% reduction) ICS/LABA combination to a fixed moderate/high-dose ICS found no significant difference in severe exacerbations requiring oral corticosteroids, withdrawal due to worsening of asthma, or airway inflammation. There were also significant improvements in FEV_1, morning and evening PEF, and percentage of rescue-free days in patients receiving ICS/LABA. In two of the studies, more participants receiving a LABA/reduced-ICS combination achieved a reduction in ICS dose. The authors

148

concluded that the addition of an LABA permits more participants on a minimum-maintenance ICS to reduce the ICS. However, the precise magnitude of the ICS-dose reduction requires further study.

ICS/LABA vs ICS Alone as First-Line Therapy

As already discussed, current guidelines recommend the addition of an LABA only in asthmatic patients who are inadequately controlled on adequate doses of an ICS. However, Ni and associates performed a systematic analysis of the results of nine randomized, controlled, clinical trials that enrolled a total of 1061 steroid-naïve adult asthmatics. Baseline FEV_1 was <80% predicted value in four trials and ≥80% in five trials. Formoterol (two trials) or salmeterol (seven trials) were added to a dose of ≤800 mcg/day of beclomethasone-equivalent of ICS (three trials) or to ≤400 mcg/day (six trials). The results showed that ICS/LABA as first-line therapy was not associated with a lower risk of exacerbations requiring oral corticosteroids than ICS alone (RR 1.2). Although FEV_1 improved significantly with ICS/LABA (weighted mean difference, 210 mL) as did symptom-free days, the change in use of rescue β-agonists was not significantly different between the groups. There was no significant group difference in adverse events, withdrawals, or withdrawals due to poor asthma control. The authors conclude that there is insufficient current evidence to recommend use of combination therapy rather than an ICS alone as a first-line treatment.

■ Fixed-Dose Combinations

Two fixed-dose combinations of an ICS and an LABA in a single dry-powder inhaler (DPI) device have been developed: salmeterol/fluticasone (Advair Diskus) and formoterol/budesonide (Symbicort). Both products are available in three different fixed-dose strengths (**Table 11.1**).

149

TABLE 11.1 — Available Strengths of Fixed-Dose Inhaled Corticosteroids and Long-Acting β-Agonists in a Single Inhaler		
Advair Diskus		
	Fluticasone	*Salmeterol*
Advair Diskus 100/50	100 mcg	50 mcg
Advair Diskus 250/50	250 mcg	50 mcg
Advair Diskus 500/50	500 mcg	50 mcg
Symbicort Turbohaler		
	Budesonide	*Formoterol*
Symbicort Turbohaler 100/6	100 mcg	6 mcg
Symbicort Turbohaler 200/6	200 mcg	6 mcg
Symbicort Turbohaler 400/6	400 mcg	6 mcg

Salmeterol/Fluticasone

Bateman and colleagues performed the first study that compared 12 weeks of treatment with the fixed-dose combination of salmeterol/fluticasone 50/100 mcg bid with the two components delivered via separate inhalers. This 12-week study in 244 patients with symptomatic asthma found no differences in clinical effects between the methods of delivery. Both treatments improved lung function measures (morning and evening PEF, FEV_1) from baseline. Both treatments were well tolerated and the prevalence of adverse events was similar in both groups.

Two subsequent 12-week studies compared the efficacy of salmeterol/fluticasone 50/100 mcg and 50/250 mcg bid with either salmeterol or fluticasone administered separately and found that the combination inhaler provided better efficacy than the same doses of the individual components alone. Kavuru and coworkers found that the mean change in FEV_1 at end point was significantly ($P \leq 0.003$) greater with the combination product (0.51 L) compared with placebo (0.01 L), salmeterol (0.11 L), and fluticasone (0.28 L) (**Figure 11.1**). In addition, the combination product significantly ($P \leq 0.012$) increased morning and evening PEF at end point compared with the other groups. Patients in the combination-product group were less likely to withdraw from the study because of worsening asthma compared with those in the other groups ($P \leq 0.020$). The fixed-dose combination significantly reduced symptom scores and rescue albuterol use compared with the other treatments and increased the percentage of nights with no awakenings and the percentage of days with no symptoms compared with placebo and salmeterol. All treatments were equally well tolerated. Similar results with salmeterol/fluticasone 50/250 mcg bid were reported by Shapiro and associates. Aubier and colleagues found that salmeterol/fluticasone 50/500 mcg bid was as effective and well tolerated in achieving asthma control in steroid-dependent patients as the separate administration of the two drugs, and both combination and concurrent therapy were superior to administration of the same dose of corticosteroid alone.

The 1-year, randomized, stratified, double-blind, parallel-group Gaining Optimal Asthma ControL (GOAL) study in 3421 patients with uncontrolled asthma compared fluticasone alone and the fixed-dose salmeterol/fluticasone combination in achieving two rigorous, composite, guideline-based measures of asthma control: total-controlled and well-controlled asthma. As defined in this study, these composite measures included asthma symptoms, lung function, and use of rescue β-agonists. Treatment was stepped-up until total control was achieved or a maximum of 500 mcg corticosteroid bid was reached. Across strata (previously corticosteroid-free, low- and moderate-dose corticosteroid users) total control was achieved by significantly ($P < 0.001$) more patients receiving

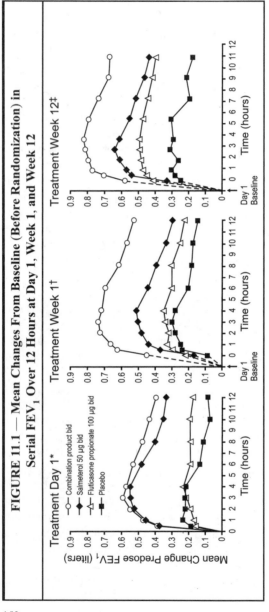

FIGURE 11.1 — Mean Changes From Baseline (Before Randomization) in Serial FEV$_1$ Over 12 Hours at Day 1, Week 1, and Week 12

Treatment Day 1*

Treatment Week 1†

Treatment Week 12‡

—○— Combination product bid
—◆— Salmeterol 50 µg bid
—△— Fluticasone propionate 100 µg bid
—■— Placebo

Mean Change Predose FEV$_1$ (liters)

Time (hours)

Day 1 Baseline

* $P < 0.001$, combination product and salmeterol *vs* placebo, all time points; $P < 0.001$ combination product *vs* fluticasone, all time points.

† $P \leq 0.05$, combination product and salmeterol *vs* placebo, all time points; $P < 0.007$ combination product *vs* salmeterol and fluticasone, all time points.

‡ $P \leq 0.039$, combination product, salmeterol, and fluticasone *vs* placebo, all time points except hours 1,3, and 6 for fluticasone; $P < 0.047$ combination product *vs* salmeterol and fluticasone, all time points.

Kavuru M, et al. *J Allergy Clin Immunol.* 2000;105:1108-1116.

11

salmeterol/fluticasone compared with those receiving fluticasone only (31% vs 19%, respectively) after dose escalation and at 1 year (41% vs 28%, respectively). Asthma became well controlled in 63% of patients with salmeterol/fluticasone compared with 50% with fluticasone (P <0.001) after dose escalation and 71% vs 59%, respectively, at 1 year. Control was achieved more rapidly and at a lower ICS dose with salmeterol/fluticasone vs fluticasone. In addition, exacerbation rates across strata (0.07–0.27 per patient per year) were significantly lower (P ≤0.009) with salmeterol/fluticasone (**Figure 11.2**). In addition, improvement in health status was significantly better with salmeterol/fluticasone.

Budesonide/Formoterol

Zetterstrom and colleagues compared the efficacy of budesonide/formoterol in a single inhaler with budesonide alone, and with concurrent administration of budesonide and formoterol from separate inhalers, in 362 adult patients with asthma not controlled with an ICS alone. In this 12-week, double-blind, double-dummy study, patients were randomized to receive single-inhaler budesonide/formoterol 160/4.5 mcg, two inhalations bid, or corresponding treatment with budesonide or budesonide plus formoterol via separate inhalers. There was a significantly (P <0.001) greater increase in morning PEF with single-inhaler and separate-inhaler budesonide and formoterol compared with budesonide alone; the effect was apparent after 1 day (**Figure 11.3**). Similarly, evening PEF (**Figure 11.3**), use of rescue medication, total asthma symptom scores, and percentage of symptom-free days improved more with both single-inhaler and separate-inhaler therapy than with budesonide alone, as did asthma control days (~15%, with a marked increase in the first week). All treatments were well tolerated and the adverse-event profile was similar in all three treatment groups.

154

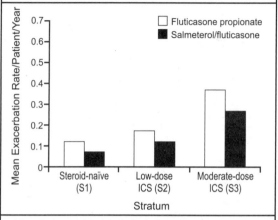

FIGURE 11.2 — Mean Rates Per Year of Exacerbations Requiring Either Oral Steroids or Hospital or Emergency Department Visits Over Weeks 1-52 Among Patients Treated With Salmeterol/Fluticasone or Fluticasone Alone

Abbreviations: ICS, inhaled corticosteroid; S, strata.

Patients stratified according to use of ICS in 6 months previous to trial enrollment.

$P \leq 0.009$ salmeterol/fluticasone vs fluticasone, all strata.

Bateman ED, et al. *Am J Respir Crit Care Med.* 2004;170:836-844.

Two subsequent studies by Rosenhall and coworkers also found equivalent efficacy and safety between the same doses of budesonide/formoterol (160/4.5 mcg, two inhalations bid), either in one inhaler or in separate inhalers, when administered for 6 or 12 months to adults with moderate persistent asthma. Furthermore, Lalloo and associates reported that in adult patients whose mild-to-moderate asthma is not fully controlled on low doses of an ICS, low-dose budesonide/formoterol (80 mcg/4.5 mcg, bid) provided greater improvements in asthma control than increasing the maintenance dose of the ICS.

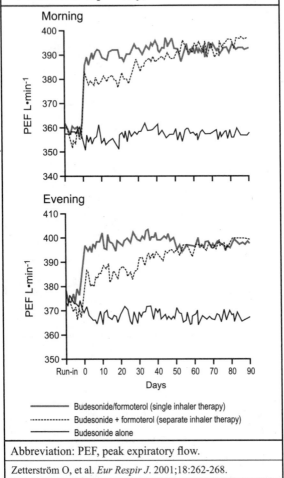

FIGURE 11.3 — Morning and Evening PEF During 12 Weeks' Treatment With Budesonide/Formoterol Single Inhaler, Budesonide Plus Formoterol Separately, or Budesonide Alone

Budesonide/formoterol (single inhaler therapy)
Budesonide + formoterol (separate inhaler therapy)
Budesonide alone

Abbreviation: PEF, peak expiratory flow.

Zetterström O, et al. *Eur Respir J*. 2001;18:262-268.

In another 12-week study, by Bateman and colleagues, 373 patients with asthma (FEV_1 78% of predicted) were randomly assigned to treatment with either budesonide/formoterol 160/4.5 mcg, one inhalation twice daily or fluticasone 250 mcg twice daily. Significantly greater increases in morning PEF, the primary efficacy variable, were observed in patients treated with budesonide/formoterol compared with fluticasone propionate (27.4 L/min vs 7.7 L/min; $P < 0.001$). Evening PEF and clinic FEV_1 also favored budesonide/formoterol compared with fluticasone propionate ($P < 0.001$), as did use of reliever medication ($P = 0.04$) and the proportion of reliever-free days ($P < 0.001$). There were also numerical improvements in symptom-free days, nighttime awakenings, and asthma-control days in favor of budesonide/formoterol. The risk of an exacerbation was reduced by 32% in the budesonide/formoterol group compared with the fluticasone propionate group ($P < 0.05$).

The long duration of action of both budesonide and formoterol suggest that the budesonide/formoterol combination could be suitable for once-daily administration. Buhl and associates randomized 523 patients with moderate persistent asthma not fully controlled with inhaled corticosteroids (400-1000 mcg/day) to receive either once-daily budesonide/formoterol (160/4.5 mcg, two inhalations), twice-daily budesonide/formoterol (160/4.5 mcg, one inhalation); or budesonide (400 mcg) once daily for 12 weeks. Once-daily dosing was administered in the evening and twice-daily dosing was administered in the morning and evening. Compared with budesonide alone, change in mean morning and evening PEF was greater in the once-daily budesonide/formoterol group ($P < 0.001$) and the twice-daily budesonide/formoterol group ($P < 0.001$). Night awakenings, symptom-free days, reliever-use–free days, and asthma-control days were all improved during once-daily budesonide/formoterol therapy vs budesonide ($P \leq 0.05$). The risk of a mild exacerbation was reduced after both once- and twice-daily budesonide/formoterol vs budesonide (38% and 35%, respectively; $P < 0.002$). The results of this study confirm those of several earlier trials that showed that once-daily budesonide/formoterol is effective in patients with mild-to-moderate and stable asthma.

A clinical trial program in more than 12,000 patients in 28 countries has assessed the efficacy of an adjustable maintenance dosing regimen with budesonide/formoterol. With this regimen, patients were treated with doses of budesonide/formoterol that were varied according to predefined criteria for asthma control. Patients also used a short-acting β-agonist for symptom relief. Those patients in whom their asthma was well controlled by budesonide/formoterol decreased their dosage to a low maintenance dose (one inhalation bid). After a period of deteriorating asthma control, defined as any of the following: 2 days with reliever medication use on three occasions during the day, nighttime awakenings, and/or a PEF value <85% of the baseline value, patients increased their dose of budesonide/formoterol from one to four inhalations bid for a period of 7 to 14 days. Once control was reestablished, the dose was once again reduced to one inhalation bid. A number of publications (see Suggested Reading at end of chapter) have reported that compared with a fixed maintenance dose of budesonide/formoterol, fewer patients in the adjustable maintenance dosing groups had exacerbations (6.2% vs 9.5%, respectively; $P < 0.05$) despite using 40% less study medications (2.35 vs 3.95 inhalations/day, respectively; $P < 0.001$). Thus better asthma control was achieved with lower doses of ICSs when patients adjusted their medication levels according to their asthma symptoms.

Inhaled Corticosteroids and Leukotriene Modifiers

The current NAEPP guidelines recommend the addition of a leukotriene modifier (see Chapter 10, *Leukotriene Modifiers*) to an ICS as an alternative to an LABA in:

- Youths ≥12 years of age and adults with mild to moderate persistent asthma unresponsive to an optimal dose of ICS
- Patients 0 to 11 years of age with mild to severe persistent asthma unresponsive to an optimal dose of ICS (in patients 0 to 4 years of age, montelukast is the only leukotriene modifier recommended for use).

A recent meta-analysis of 27 (25 adult and 2 pediatric) randomized, placebo-controlled trials by Ducharme and associates found that in symptomatic asthmatic patients, the addition of approved doses of leukotriene modifiers to ICSs resulted in a nonsignificant reduction in the risk of exacerbations requiring systemic steroids (RR 0.64). However, there was a modest improvement in PEF (mean difference, 7.7 L/min) together with a decrease in the use of rescue short-acting β-agonist (mean difference 1 puff/week). In ICS-sparing studies of patients who were well controlled at baseline, addition of a leukotriene modifier produced no overall difference in dose of inhaled glucocorticoids (mean difference –21 mcg/d), but it was associated with fewer withdrawals due to poor asthma control. The authors concluded that the addition of approved doses of leukotriene modifiers as add-on therapy to inhaled glucocorticoids results in modest improvement in lung function.

Several studies have compared the efficacy of adding a leukotriene modifier or an LABA to ICS

11

therapy in symptomatic patients with moderate or severe persistent asthma. The double-blind study by Ilowite and coworkers randomized 1473 patients to receive salmeterol (84 mcg/d) or montelukast (10 mg/d) as add-on to inhaled fluticasone (220 mcg/d) for 48 weeks. Eighty percent of patients in the montelukast group and 83.3% of patients in the salmeterol group remained free of exacerbations during the 48 weeks of treatment (RR 1.20) Treatment with montelukast significantly reduced blood eosinophil counts compared with salmeterol, whereas salmeterol significantly increased pre-albuterol FEV_1, asthma-specific quality of life, and morning PEF and decreased nocturnal awakenings compared with montelukast. The authors noted that while the addition of montelukast or salmeterol to an ICS similarly protected most patients from experiencing an exacerbation during a 1-year period; based on noninferiority limits, the study was inconclusive with regard to a difference between treatment groups.

A small study in 40 symptomatic patients with moderately persistent asthma using 400 mcg/day budesonide, Ceylan and colleagues added inhaled formoterol (9 mcg) twice a day in 20 patients and oral montelukast (10 mg) once daily for 8 weeks. There was a significantly (P <0.05) greater increase from baseline in morning PEF in formoterol-treated patients than in those receiving montelukast (54.2 L/min vs 30.5 L/min, respectively). The increase from baseline in nighttime PEF was also significantly greater in formoterol-treated patients (44.5 L/min vs 27 L/min, respectively; P <0.001). In addition, increases in asthma symptom scores and reductions in the use of rescue medication were significantly greater in patients receiving add-on formoterol than in those receiving add-on montelukast (P <0.0001 for both measures).

Another small, 6-week study by Tsuchida and associates compared the additive effects of a leukotriene modifier (pranlukast 450 mg/day) and a sustained-release theophylline (200 mg/day) with a moderate dose of ICS (beclomethasone 800 mcg/day) on PEF and asthma-related symptoms. Neither combined regimen significantly changed symptom scores or the use of rescue medication, although both agents significantly increased morning and evening PEF compared with the ICS-only run-in period.

Inhaled Corticosteroid and Theophylline

Recent studies have suggested that theophylline may exert anti-inflammatory and immunomodulatory effects as well as a steroid-sparing effect. Currently, addition of a sustained-release oral theophylline (to a serum concentration of 5 to 15 mcg/mL) to an ICS is another alternative combination regimen recommended in the NAEPP guidelines. A recent randomized, open, parallel-group trial by Wang and colleagues compared the effects the combination of a slow-release theophylline (200 mg/day) and inhaled beclomethasone (250 mcg bid) with beclomethasone (500 mcg bid) alone, on asthma control and anti-inflammatory activity in 41 adult asthma patients. At the start and at the end of the 6-week treatment period, lung function testing and sputum induction were performed, and plasma cortisol levels were measured. Sputum was analyzed for cell differential counts and interleukin (IL)-5 levels. Compared with baseline, both the combination of ICS and theophylline and double-dose ICS had similar beneficial effects on asthma control, symptom score, and lung function. Both therapies had similar airway anti-inflammatory effects. The authors suggest that combining theophylline with ICS may allow a reduction in ICS dose.

Inhaled Corticosteroid and Anti-IgE Antibody

As discussed in Chapter 13, *Anti-IgE Therapy*, the humanized, murine anti-IgE antibody omalizumab represents a novel and efficacious form of add-on therapy for patients with allergic asthma. Numerous clinical trials have demonstrated significant benefits in terms of reducing exacerbations in patients with moderate-to-severe persistent asthma. In addition, adding omalizumab to an ICS can result in significant reductions in the doses of steroids. Furthermore, omalizumab appears to be safe and well tolerated and may improve patient quality of life. Although omalizumab is recommended to be considered as an add-on in youths ≥12 years of age and adults in the current NAEPP guidelines, it is indicated for a specific population of patients with documented allergic asthma. The relative inconvenience of monthly or biweekly subcutaneous injections and a cost typical of many biologic agents can limit its widespread use.

Combination Therapy for Persistent Asthma: Summary

Inhaled corticosteroids are the foundation of maintenance therapy for persistent asthma. However, many eventually require either an increased dose of ICS or the addition of one or more other medications to maintain satisfactory control of their symptoms. Considerable clinical trial evidence has demonstrated the efficacy and safety of an LABA as the first add-on agent. Other medications, including cromolyn, nedocromil, leukotriene modifiers, sustained-release theophylline, and omalizumab in allergic asthma can be considered alternative choices for combination therapy in selected patients. The recent availability of combinations of an ICS and an LABA administered via a single inhaler provide convenience and facilitate adherence.

SUGGESTED READING

Aalbers R, Backer V, Kava TT, et al. Adjustable maintenance dosing with budesonide/formoterol compared with fixed-dose salmeterol/fluticasone in moderate to severe asthma. *Curr Med Res Opin.* 2004;20:225-240.

Ankerst J. Combination inhalers containing inhaled corticosteroids and long-acting beta2-agonists: improved clinical efficacy and dosing options in patients with asthma. *J Asthma.* 2005;42:715-724.

Aubier M, Pieters WR, Schlosser NJ, Steinmetz KO. Salmeterol/fluticasone propionate (50/500 microg) in combination in a Diskus inhaler (Seretide) is effective and safe in the treatment of steroid-dependent asthma. *Respir Med.* 1999;93:876-884.

Bateman ED, Bantje TA, Joao Gomes M, et al. Combination therapy with single inhaler budesonide/formoterol compared with high dose of fluticasone propionate alone in patients with moderate persistent asthma. *Am J Respir Med.* 2003;2:275-281.

Bateman ED, Britton M, Almeida J, et al. Salmeterol/fluticasone combination inhaler. A new, effective, and well-tolerated treatment for asthma. *Clin Drug Investig.* 1998;16:193-210.

Bateman ED, Boushey HA, Bousquet J, et al: GOAL Investigators Group. Can guideline-defined asthma control be achieved? The Gaining Optimal Asthma ControL study. *Am J Respir Crit Care Med.* 2004;170:836-844.

Buhl R, Creemers JP, Vondra V, Martelli NA, Naya IP, Ekstrom T. Once-daily budesonide/formoterol in a single inhaler in adults with moderate persistent asthma. *Respir Med.* 2003;97:323-330.

Ceylan E, Gencer M, Aksoy S. Addition of formoterol or montelukast to low-dose budesonide: an efficacy comparison in short- and long-term asthma control. *Respiration.* 2004;71:594-601.

Currie GP, Lee DK, Srivastava P. Long-acting bronchodilator or leukotriene modifier as add-on therapy to inhaled corticosteroids in persistent asthma? *Chest.* 2005;128:2954-2962.

11

Ducharme F, Schwartz Z, Hicks G, Kakuma R. Addition of anti-leukotriene agents to inhaled corticosteroids for chronic asthma. *Cochrane Database Syst Rev.* 2004;(2):CD003133.

FitzGerald JM, Sears MR, Boulet LP, et al; Canadian Investigators. Adjustable maintenance dosing with budesonide/formoterol reduces asthma exacerbations compared with traditional fixed dosing: a five-month multicenter Canadian study. *Can Respir J.* 2003;10:427-434.

Foresi A, Morelli MC, Catena E; on behalf of the Italian Study Group. Low-dose budesonide with the addition of an increased dose during exacerbations is effective in long-term asthma control. *Chest.* 2000;117:440-446.

Gibson PG, Powell H, Ducharme F. Long-acting beta2-agonists as an inhaled corticosteroid-sparing agent for chronic asthma in adults and children. *Cochrane Database Syst Rev.* 2005 Oct 19;(4):CD005076.

Greenstone IR, Ni Chroinin MN, Masse V, et al. Combination of inhaled long-acting beta2-agonists and inhaled steroids versus higher dose of inhaled steroids in children and adults with persistent asthma. *Cochrane Database Syst Rev.* 2005 Oct 19;(4):CD005533.

Ilowite J, Webb R, Friedman B, et al. Addition of montelukast or salmeterol to fluticasone for protection against asthma attacks: a randomized, double-blind, multicenter study. *Ann Allergy Asthma Immunol.* 2004;92:641-648.

Kavuru M, Melamed J, Gross G, et al. Salmeterol and fluticasone propionate combined in a new powder inhalation device for the treatment of asthma: a randomized, double-blind, placebo-controlled trial. *J Allergy Clin Immunol.* 2000;105:1108-1116.

Koopmans JG, Lutter R, Jansen HM, van der Zee JS. Adding salmeterol to an inhaled corticosteroid: long-term effects on bronchial inflammation in asthma. *Thorax.* 2006;61(4):306-312.

Lalloo UG, Malolepszy J, Kozma D, et al. Budesonide and formoterol in a single inhaler improves asthma control compared with increasing the dose of corticosteroid in adults with mild-to-moderate asthma. *Chest.* 2003;123:1480-1487.

Leuppi JD, Salzberg M, Meyer L, et al. An individualized, adjustable maintenance regimen of budesonide/formoterol provides effective asthma symptom control at a lower overall dose than fixed dosing. *Swiss Med Wkly.* 2003;133:302-309.

Masoli M, Weatherall M, Holt S, Beasley R. Moderate dose inhaled corticosteroids plus salmeterol versus higher doses of inhaled corticosteroids in symptomatic asthma. *Thorax.* 2005;60:730-734.

Ni Chroinin M, Greenstone IR, Danish A, et al. Long-acting beta2-agonists versus placebo in addition to inhaled corticosteroids in children and adults with chronic asthma. *Cochrane Database Syst Rev.* 2005 Oct 19;(4):CD005535.

Ni CM, Greenstone IR, Ducharme FM. Addition of inhaled long-acting beta2-agonists to inhaled steroids as first line therapy for persistent asthma in steroid-naive adults. *Cochrane Database Syst Rev.* 2005 Apr 18;(2):CD005307.

O'Byrne PM, Bisgaard H, Godard PP, et al. Budesonide/formoterol combination therapy as both maintenance and reliever medication in asthma. *Am J Respir Crit Care Med.* 2005;171:129-136.

Reynolds NA, Lyseng-Williamson KA, Wiseman LR. Inhaled salmeterol/fluticasone propionate: a review of its use in asthma. *Drugs.* 2005;65:1715-1734.

Rosenhall L, Elvstrand A, Tilling B, et al. One-year safety and efficacy of budesonide/formoterol in a single inhaler (Symbicort Turbuhaler) for the treatment of asthma. *Respir Med.* 2003;97:702-708.

Rosenhall L, Heinig JH, Lindqvist A, Leegaard J, Stahl E, Bergqvist PB. Budesonide/formoterol (Symbicort) is well tolerated and effective in patients with moderate persistent asthma. *Int J Clin Pract.* 2002;56:427-433.

Shapiro G, Lumry W, Wolfe J, et al. Combined salmeterol 50 microg and fluticasone propionate 250 microg in the diskus device for the treatment of asthma. *Am J Respir Crit Care Med.* 2000;161:527-534.

Sin DD, Man SF. Corticosteroids and adrenoceptor agonists: the compliments for combination therapy in chronic airways diseases. *Eur J Pharmacol.* 2006;533:28-35.

11

Stallberg B, Olsson P, Jorgensen LA, Lindarck N, Ekstrom T. Budes-onide/formoterol adjustable maintenance dosing reduces asthma ex-acerbations versus fixed dosing. *Int J Clin Pract*. 2003;57:656-661.

Tsuchida T, Matsuse H, Machida I, et al. Evaluation of theophylline or pranlukast, a cysteinyl leukotriene receptor 1 antagonist, as add-on therapy in uncontrolled asthmatic patients with a medium dose of inhaled corticosteroids. *Allergy Asthma Proc*. 2005;26:287-291.

Wang Y, Wang CZ, Lin KX, et al. Comparison of inhaled corticoster-oid combined with theophylline and double-dose inhaled corticoster-oid in moderate to severe asthma. *Respirology*. 2005;10:189-195.

Zetterstrom O, Buhl R, Mellem H, et al. Improved asthma control with budesonide/formoterol in a single inhaler, compared with budes-onide alone. *Eur Respir J*. 2001;18:262-268.

12 Inhalation Devices

Inhaled bronchodilators and corticosteroids are the mainstays of the treatment of asthma. A variety of devices, including nebulizers, pressurized metered-dose inhalers (MDI), and dry-powder inhalers (DPI), are currently available. However, in the United States, not all approved medications are available for administration via all inhaler systems (**Table 12.1** and **Table 12.2**). Thus the sheer number of options may be confusing when choosing the best one for an individual patient. Fortunately, clinical evidence shows that most of these devices will work for most clinical situations, *when used correctly*. The physician must consider a number of factors when choosing a drug/device combination for a patient. These include the cognitive and physical ability of the patient, ease of use, convenience, cost, and patient preference. Once the decision has been made, detailed education of the patient (or parent, in the case of a child) on the proper use of the device is critical. To assess ongoing adherence, the patient should be requested to demonstrate how they use the device. This is a particularly important step when a patient reports that the medication "doesn't seem to be working."

Errors in Inhaler Use

Patient errors in using their inhaler device are quite common. Several studies have documented poor knowledge and technique both in patients and in caregivers. In the largest study of patient inhaler technique, Molimard and colleagues observed over 3800 outpatients treated for at least 1 month with their prescribed inhalant devices (both MDIs and DPIs). Approximately

167

Drug	Nebulizer	MDI	Breath-Actuated	DPI Single-Dose	DPI Multi-Dose
Albuterol	Yes	Yes*	No	No	No
Levalbuterol	Yes	Yes*	No	No	No
Pirbuterol	No	No	Yes	No	No
Ipratropium[†]	Yes	Yes	No	No	No
Albuterol + ipratropium[†]	Yes	Yes	No	No	No
Salmeterol	No	No	No	No	Yes
Formoterol	No	No	No	Yes	No
Tiotropium[†]	No	No	No	Yes	No

TABLE 12.1 — Inhaled Bronchodilator Device Combinations Available in the United States

Abbreviations: DPI, dry-powder inhaler; MDI, metered-dose inhaler.

* Available in hydrofluoralkane (HFA) formulation.

[†] Not currently approved for asthma.

Geller DE. *Respir Care.* 2005;50:1313–1321.

TABLE 12.2 — Inhaled Corticosteroid Device Combinations Available in the United States

Drug	Nebulizer	MDI	Breath-Actuated	DPI Single-Dose	DPI Multi-Dose
Beclomethasone	No	Yes*	No	No	No
Budesonide	Yes	No	No	No	Yes
Budesonide/formoterol	No	Yes†	No	No	No
Ciclesonide	No	Yes†	No	No	No
Flunisolide	No	Yes†	No	No	No
Fluticasone	No	Yes*	No	No	No
Fluticasone/salmeterol	No	Yes†	No	No	Yes
Mometasone	No	No	No	No	Yes
Triamcinolone	No	Yes	No	No	No

Abbreviations: DPI, dry-powder inhaler; MDI, metered-dose inhaler.

* Available in hydrofluoralkane (HFA) formulation.
† HFA formulation in development.

Geller DE. *Respir Care.* 2005;50:1313-1321.

12

half of the patients made at least one error when using their MDI or DPI. Among those using an MDI, 76% made at least one error. Critical errors that would result in almost no medication reaching the lungs were made by 11% of those using a DPI and 28% of those using an MDI. These results, and those of many other studies, underline the critical need for more education of patients on proper use of inhaled asthma medications.

Device Advantages and Disadvantages

Every type of inhaler has advantages and disadvantages relative to other types that must be considered in the selection of a device for a particular patient. A recent comprehensive review of the clinical trial literature by Dolovich and associates identified the advantages and disadvantages of each type of device (**Table 12.3**).

■ Nebulizers

No special technique or patient coordination is required for the use of a nebulizer. However, preparation, medication administration, and device cleaning take considerably longer than with an MDI or DPI. Furthermore, the performance efficiency of different nebulizers can be variable, depending on many factors. In general, nebulizers are often used with small children and in the emergency department and inpatient settings.

■ Metered-Dose Inhalers

The pressurized MDI has a number of advantages. **Figure 12.1** illustrates two types of MDIs: a chlorofluorocarbon (CFC)-propelled MDI and a breath-powered, dry-powder MDI. Such devices are small, portable, and can be used very quickly. As can be seen in **Table 12.1** and **Table 12.2**, more medications are currently available in an MDI than any other type of device. However, proper MDI technique is critical for optimal inhaled drug delivery (**Figure 12.2** and **Figure 12.3**). Many studies suggest that patients often do not use MDIs properly. For example, if there is a delay between actuation and inhalation, or if the patient inhales too quickly, drug delivery to the lower airways will be affected.

In general, the open-mouth method is preferred to the closed-mouth method to minimize posterior pharyngeal side effects as well as to maximize drug deposition in the distal tracheobronchial tree. The critical steps of the open-mouth method include:

- Shake the canister
- Place the canister two finger-breadths from the lips
- With the mouth open, actuate the MDI at the beginning of a tidal inspiration
- Close the mouth and hold breath for 10 seconds.

The open-mouth method (**Figure 12.2**) should be attempted in cooperative patients who may be able to master the technique (ie, patients who do not have arthritis, tremor, etc). If a patient cannot demonstrate adequate MDI technique by the open-mouth method, a spacer device should be routinely used. Commonly used spacer devices are shown in **Figure 12.4**. Commercially available spacers include:

- Ace Aerosol Cloud Enhancer (**Figure 12.5**)
- AeroChamber (**Figure 12.6**)
- InspirEase (**Figure 12.7**)
- OptiHaler (**Figure 12.8**).

The environmental impact of CFC (freon) used in pressurized MDIs has received much recent attention. Most MDIs contain a blend of CFC propellants, including CFC-12 (primary propellant), CFC-11 (pri-

TABLE 12.3 — Advantages and Disadvantages of Currently Available Inhalation Devices

Type	Advantages	Disadvantages
Small-volume jet nebulizer	• Patient coordination required • Effective with tidal breathing • Lengthy treatment time • High dose possible • Dose modification possible • No CFC release • Can be used with supplemental oxygen • Can deliver combination therapies if compatible	• Lack of portability (pressurized gas source required) • Lengthy treatment time • Device cleaning required • Contamination possible • Not all medication available in solution form • Does not aerosolize suspensions well • Device preparation required • Performance variability • Expensive when compressor added in
Ultrasonic nebulizer	• Patient coordination not required • High dose possible • Dose modification possible • No CFC release • Small dead volume • Quiet • Newer designs small and portable	• Expensive • Need for electrical power source (wall outlet or batteries) • Contamination possible • Not all medication available in solution form • Device preparation required before treatment • Does not nebulize suspensions well • Possible drug degradation

	• Faster delivery than jet nebulizer • No drug loss during exhalation (breath-actuated devices)	• Potential for airway irritation with some drugs
Pressurized MDI	• Portable and compact • Treatment time is short • No drug preparation required • No contamination of contents • Dose-dose reproducibility high • Some can be used with breath-actuated mouthpiece	• Coordination of breathing and actuation needed • Device actuation required • High pharyngeal deposition • Upper limit to unit dose content • Remaining doses difficult to determine • Potential for abuse • Not all medications available • Many use CFC propellants in United States
Holding chamber, reverse-flow spacer, or spacer	• Reduces need for patient coordination • Reduces pharyngeal deposition	• Inhalation can be more complex for some patients • Can reduce dose available if not used properly • More expensive than MDI alone • Less portable than MDI alone • Integral actuator devices may alter aerosol properties

Continued

12

DPI	• Breath-actuated • Less patient coordination required • Propellant not required • Small and portable • Short treatment time • Dose counters in most newer designs	• Requires moderate to high inspiratory flow • Some units are single dose • Can result in high pharyngeal deposition • Not all medications available

Abbreviations: CFC, chlorofluorocarbon; DPI, dry-powder inhaler; MDI, metered-dose inhaler.

Adapted from: Dolovich MB et al. *Chest.* 2005; 127:335-371.

FIGURE 12.1 — Representative Metered-Dose Inhalers

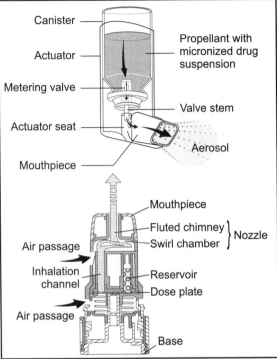

Top: Schematic diagram of a typical chlorofluorocarbon-propelled metered-dose inhaler. A dose of propellant containing the suspended particles of drug enters the metering valve. When the canister is pushed down, the contents of the valve are released through the valve stem and escape from the actuator seat as a fine aerosol. *Bottom:* Schematic diagram of the Twisthaler (Schering-Plough), which is representative of the breath-actuated, dry-powder, metered-dose inhalers. Twisting the cap in a counterclockwise direction and removing it delivers a dose of finely powdered drug from the drug reservoir to the inhalation channel. When the patient breathes in through the mouthpiece, the powder passes through the mouthpiece and is administered to the patient. Other examples of breath-actuated, dry-powder, metered-dose inhalers include the Aerolizer (Schering-Plough), Diskus (GlaxoSmithKline), and Turbuhaler (AstraZeneca).

Modified from: Nelson HS. *N Engl J Med.* 1995;333:501.

FIGURE 12.2 — Use of Metered-Dose Inhaler: Open-Mouth Technique

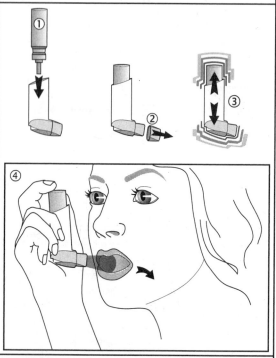

1) Insert metal vial into plastic oral adapter; *2)* Remove dust cap from oral adapter and inspect for foreign objects; *3)* Shake inhaler well; *4)* Breathe out fully, positioning mouth-piece of oral adapter two finger-breadths in front of opened mouth. Begin to breathe in deeply while pressing the vial firmly down into the adapter with the index finger, releasing one metered dose. Release pressure on the vial, moving it away from mouth. Hold breath for 10 seconds, then breathe out slowly. Begin with a single dose; repeat process for second inhalation. Replace dust cap after each use.

FIGURE 12.3 — Use of Metered-Dose Inhaler: Maxair Autohaler

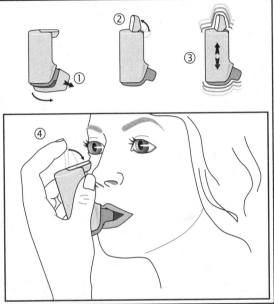

1) Remove mouthpiece cover by pulling down lip on back of cover, and inspect mouthpiece for foreign objects; *2)* While holding autohaler in upright position, raise lever so that it stays up; it will "snap" into place; *3)* Shake gently several times; *4)* Exhale normally before use. Seal lips around mouthpiece of Maxair Autohaler, inhaling deeply with steady, moderate force. An audible "click" will be heard as the lever snaps down automatically. Continue to take a full, deep breath. Remove autohaler from mouth and hold breath for 10 seconds then exhale slowly. If physician has prescribed additional puffs, wait 1 minute then repeat step 4. Replace mouthpiece cover after each use.

12

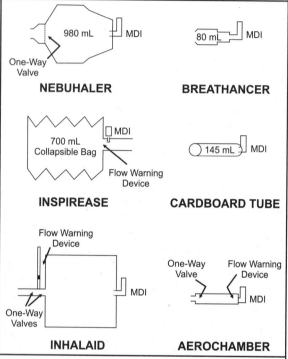

FIGURE 12.4 — Schematic Depiction of Six Commonly Used Metered-Dose Inhaler Spacer Devices

Abbreviation: MDI, metered-dose inhaler.

Modified from: *Bronchial Asthma: Mechanisms and Therapeutics.* 3rd ed. Weiss EB, Stein M, eds. Boston, Mass: Little Brown & Co; 1993:751.

FIGURE 12.5 — Use of Metered-Dose Inhaler With Spacer: ACE Aerosol Cloud Enhancer

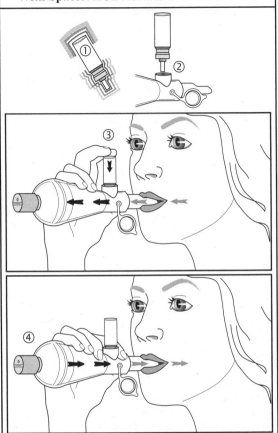

1) Shake metered-dose inhaler (MDI) canister well; *2)* Place the MDI canister stem into the canister port of the ACE Aerosol Cloud Enhancer dispenser; *3)* Place the mouthpiece between the teeth, closing lips around it. Exhale normally then press down firmly on the canister; *4)* Take a slow, deep breath through the mouthpiece, being careful not to breathe in so quickly as to activate the flow signal whistle. Hold breath for 10 seconds. Remove the inhaler from mouth and exhale slowly. If physician has instructed more than one puff, wait 1 or 2 minutes, then repeat steps 1 through 4.

FIGURE 12.6 — Use of Metered-Dose Inhaler With Spacer: AeroChamber

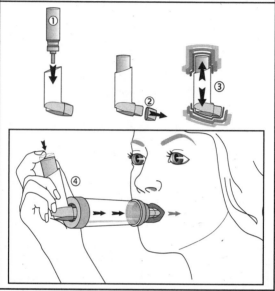

1) Insert metal vial into metered-dose inhaler (MDI); *2)* Remove dust cap from MDI and inspect for foreign objects; *3)* Shake MDI well; *4)* Insert MDI mouthpiece into the round opening in the rubber-like ring at the end of the AeroChamber. Exhale normally. Place the AeroChamber mouthpiece in mouth and close lips. Depress metal vial to spray only one puff from the MDI into the AeroChamber. Take a slow, deep breath through the mouthpiece, being careful not to breathe so quickly as to activate the flow signal whistle. Hold breath for 10 seconds, repeating steps 1 through 4 as prescribed by physician.

FIGURE 12.7 — Use of Metered-Dose Inhaler With Spacer: InspirEase

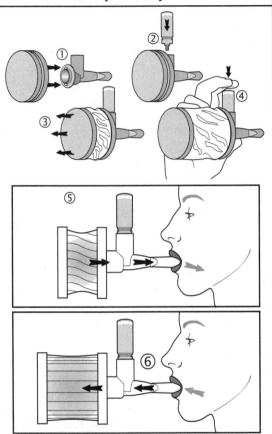

1) Connect mouthpiece to the reservoir bag, lining up locking tabs, pushing in and twisting to lock; *2)* Shake metered-dose inhaler (MDI) well then place its stem in the mouthpiece; *3)* Untwist the reservoir bag gently to open it to its full size; *4)* Place mouthpiece in mouth, closing lips tightly around it. Depress MDI with fingers, placing thumb under mouthpiece and releasing one dose; *5)* Breathe in slowly through mouthpiece careful not to breathe so quickly as to activate the flow signal whistle. Breathe in until the bag collapses. Hold breath and count to 10; *6)* Breathe out slowly into the bag. Repeat actuation as prescribed.

FIGURE 12.8 — Use of Metered-Dose Inhaler With Spacer: OptiHaler

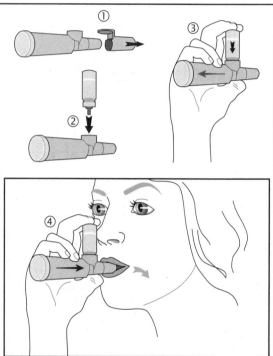

1) Remove dust cap from OptiHaler drug delivery appa-
ratus, checking for foreign objects; *2)* Insert medication
canister into OptiHaler; *3)* Depress canister which directs
medication particles away from the mouth into the chamber where they mix with incoming air; *4)* Exhale breath
before use. Seal lips around OptiHaler mouthpiece, inhale
deeply, and hold breath for 10 seconds. Remove OptiHaler
from mouth, replacing dust cap.

mary solvent), and CFC-114 (moderates pressure and density). A number of international conferences have been held that have resulted in an agreement to ban the use of CFCs after 1998-1999, including medical use. As a result, a number of pharmaceutical companies have responded to this challenge by developing new inhalers that do not use CFCs. One strategy has been to utilize a non-CFC propellant, such as hydrofluoralkane (HFA) formulations.

■ **Dry-Powder Inhalers**

DPIs are the newest type of inhaler device. These devices come in many forms, from single-dose devices that use drug contained in a capsule (eg, Turbohaler), multidose devices with bulk medication and a dosing chamber, and multidose devices with individual doses inside (eg, Diskus).

In addition to being environmentally safe, the breath-actuated DPIs do not require the exact patient coordination and synchronization typically necessary for MDI use. Also, the powder preparations can be inhaled without the need for a spacer extension device. However, these devices require a minimum inspiratory flow rate from a spontaneously breathing patient, and their use may sometimes cause throat irritation.

12

SUGGESTED READING

Ahrens RC. The role of MDI and DPI in pediatric patients: "Children are not just miniature adults." *Respir Care*. 2005;50:1323-1328.

Anderson PJ. History of aerosol therapy: liquid nebulization to MDIs to DPIs. *Respir Care*. 2005;50:1139-1149.

Capriotti T. Changes in inhaler devices for asthma and COPD. *Medsurg Nurs*. 2005;14:185-194.

Cates C. Spacers and nebulisers for the delivery of β-agonists in non-life-threatening acute asthma. *Respir Med*. 2003;97:762-769.

Cates CC, Bara A, Crilly JA, et al. Holding chambers versus nebulizers for β-agonist treatment of acute asthma. *Cochrane Database Syst Rev*. 2003;(3):CD000052.

Dolovich M, MacIntyre NR, Anderson PJ, et al. Consensus statement: aerosols and delivery devices. American Association for Respiratory Care. *Respir Care*. 2000;45:589-596.

Dolovich MB, Ahrens RC, Hess DR, et al. Device selection and outcomes of aerosol therapy: evidence-based guidelines. *Chest*. 2005;127:335-371.

Geller DE. Comparing clinical features of the nebulizer, metered-dose inhaler, and dry-powder inhaler. *Respir Care*. 2005;50:1313-1321.

Molimard M, Raherison C, Lignot S, et al. Assessment of handling of inhaler devices in real life: an observational study in 3811 patients in primary care. *J Aerosol Med*. 2003;16:249-254.

13   Anti-IgE Therapy

IgE and Asthma

It is widely, but not universally, held than asthma can be divided into allergic and nonallergic types. A major difference between these two is the presence and etiologic role of allergen-specific immunoglobulin (IgE) antibodies. A direct correlation between serum IgE levels and asthma has been demonstrated. For example, asthma prevalence increases linearly as log IgE values increase, even in patients considered to have nonallergic asthma.

Allergen-specific IgE molecules may cause airway inflammation in asthma through activation of mast cells and basophils via binding to, and cross-linking, high-affinity (FcεRI) cell-surface IgE receptors. Activation of these effector cells results in degranulation and release of inflammatory mediators, such as histamine, leukotrienes, and tumor necrosis factor alpha (TNFα), which can cause the symptoms of asthma.

Recent advances in the understanding of the role of IgE in the etiology of allergic inflammation have led to the development of omalizumab (Xolair), a humanized, murine monoclonal antibody (mAb) to IgE that has been shown to reduce serum IgE levels, and consequently, allergic inflammation. Omalizumab is currently indicated for adults and adolescents (12 years of age and older) with moderate-to-severe persistent asthma who also have a positive skin test or *in vitro* reactivity to a perennial aeroallergen, and whose symptoms are inadequately controlled with inhaled corticosteroids (ICSs).

Mechanism of Action

Omalizumab binds free (unbound) IgE in the serum regardless of allergen specificity (**Figure 13.1**). The bound IgE cannot bind to the high-affinity FcεRI receptor on mast cells and basophils because omalizumab binds to the same region on the IgE molecule by which it binds to the FcεRI receptor. Omalizumab does not bind to IgE already bound to the FcεRI receptor, which could lead to mast cell degranulation by cross-linking the receptor. In addition, omalizumab indirectly downregulates the number of Fcε-RI receptors on the surface of basophils, thereby reducing the cell's ability to degranulate.

Clinical Studies

Early clinical studies in patients with mild allergic asthma found that treatment with omalizumab significantly attenuated both early- and late-phase responses to airway challenge with specific allergens. There were reductions in the magnitude of the decreases in forced expiratory volume in 1 second (FEV_1) and a 2-fold increase in the concentration of allergen required to induce bronchoconstriction. After 8 weeks of treatment, omalizumab decreased sputum eosinophils both before and after allergen challenge. These early studies suggested that treatment with omalizumab may provide a benefit in allergic asthma by attenuating the early and late asthmatic response to allergens.

These early studies were followed by a placebo-controlled phase 2 clinical trial in 317 patients with moderate-to-severe asthma that compared the effect of omalizumab administered intravenously in low and high doses on daily asthma symptoms and oral corticosteroid doses. The daily asthma symptom score improved significantly by 42% in the high-dose group

FIGURE 13.1 — Proposed Mechanisms of Action of Omalizumab

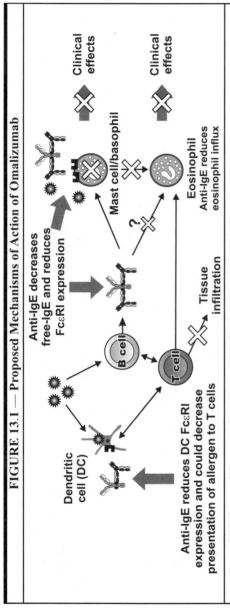

Omalizumab binds to and decreases free immunoglobulin E (IgE) levels and reduces FcεRI receptor expression on mast cells and basophils, which results in decreased mast cell activation and sensitivity, which leads to a reduction of eosinophil influx and activation. Omalizumab also reduces dendritic cell FcεRI receptor expression. Anti-IgE treatment with omalizumab might also result in decreased mast cell survival.

Holgate S, et al. *J Allergy Clin Immunol.* 2005;115:459-465.

compared with 30% with placebo. In addition, a 50% reduction in oral corticosteroid dose was seen in 78% of patients in the high-dose group compared with 33% in the placebo group.

Subsequently, three randomized, placebo-controlled phase 3 trials of similar design evaluated the effects of subcutaneous omalizumab dosed according to baseline IgE level and body weight (at least 0.016 mg/kg/IgE [IU/mL] every 4 weeks) in patients aged 12 to 76 years with moderate-to-severe asthma. Patients were required to have a baseline IgE level between 30 and 700 IU/mL and a body weight of no more than 150 kg. After initial screening, patients were converted to a common ICS (beclomethasone in two studies and fluticasone in the third) for a 4- to 6-week run-in period. Patients were then randomized to receive subcutaneous treatment with either omalizumab or placebo for a total of 28 weeks. The first 16 weeks represented the steroid-stable phase during which the steroid dose was unchanged unless an acute exacerbation required a dose increase. This period was followed by a 12- or 16-week steroid reduction phase. The end points in these studies were asthma exacerbations during the stable steroid and steroid-reduction phases, and the proportion of patients in which the dose of ICS was reduced.

As shown in **Table 13.1**, in two of these studies, the number of exacerbations per patient was significantly reduced in patients treated with omalizumab compared with placebo.

In the study by Busse and colleagues, the proportion of patients who were able to reduce their dose of beclomethasone by at least 50% was significantly greater with omalizumab treatment than with placebo (median 75% vs 50% [P <0.001]), and complete discontinuation of beclomethasone was more likely with omalizumab (39.6% vs 19.1% [P <0.001]). Improvements in asthma symptoms and pulmonary function occurred along with a reduction in rescue

TABLE 13.1 — Frequency of Exacerbations per Patient in Two Phase 3 Clinical Trials

Exacerbations/Patient	Busse et al 2001		Soler et al 2001	
	Omalizumab *n*=268 (%)	Placebo *n*=257 (%)	Omalizumab *n*=274 (%)	Placebo *n*=272 (%)
Stable Steroid Phase (16 wks)				
0	85.8	76.7	87.6	69.9
1	11.9	16.7	11.3	25.0
≥2	2.2	6.6	1.1	5.1
P value	0.005		<0.001	
Mean number of exacerbations/patient	0.2	0.3	0.1	0.4
Steroid Reduction Phase (12 weeks)				
0	78.7	67.7	83.9	70.2
1	19.0	28.4	14.2	26.1
≥2	2.2	3.9	1.8	3.7
P value	0.004		<0.001	
Mean number of exacerbations/patient	0.2	0.4	0.2	0.3

Busse W, et al. *J Allergy Clinn Immunol.* 2001;108:184-190; Soler M, et al. *Eur Respir J.* 2001;18:254-261.

13

β-agonist use. In their study, Soler and associates found that 79% of omalizumab patients were able to reduce their dose of beclomethasone by at least 50% and 43% were able to discontinue their ICSs completely as compared with 55% and 9% of placebo-treated patients, respectively.

Although the third phase 3 study by Holgate and colleagues used a similar design, the study population was somewhat different in that the 251 patients had severe persistent asthma and were stabilized on high doses of fluticasone ($\geq$1000 mcg/d). The primary endpoint was reduction in ICS dose. The results showed that 73.8% of patients in the omalizumab group and 50.8% of patients in the placebo group achieved a $\geq$50% reduction in fluticasone dose ($P = 0.001$) and the fluticasone dose was reduced to $\leq$500 mcg/day in 60.3% of omalizumab recipients vs 45.8% of placebo-treated patients ($P = 0.026$). Although there was a trend toward fewer exacerbations per patient in the omalizumab group compared with the placebo group, it did not reach significance since the study was not powered to assess this outcome. Through both phases of the trial, omalizumab reduced rescue medication requirements and improved asthma symptoms and asthma-related quality of life compared with placebo.

Patients who completed one of the 28-week studies were enrolled in a 24-week double-blind extension phase to assess the effect of omalizumab on long-term control in patients with severe allergic asthma. During the extension phase, patients were maintained on randomized treatment (omalizumab or placebo) and the lowest sustainable dose of beclomethasone. The use of other asthma medications was permitted during the extension phase. A total of 460 patients (omalizumab, n=245; placebo, n=215) entered the extension phase. Overall, omalizumab-treated patients experienced significantly fewer exacerbations vs placebo during the extension phase (0.60 and 0.83 exacerbations per patient, respectively; $P = 0.023$), despite a sustained significant reduction in their use of ICSs (mean beclomethasone equivalent dose: omalizumab, 227 mcg/d; placebo, 335 mcg/d; $P < 0.001$).

Holgate and associates performed a pooled analysis of a subgroup of 254 adolescent and adult patients at high risk for asthma-related morbidity and mortality who participated in one of the three phase 3 studies and found that the annualized rate of significant exacerbations was reduced by 50% in patients who received omalizumab compared with those who received placebo (mean rates/patient 0.69 vs 1.56, respectively, $P = 0.007$). Another pooled analysis of 1405 patients from the phase 3 trials by Corren and coworkers evaluated the rates of serious exacerbations that required hospitalization, unscheduled outpatient visits, or emergency department treatments. The incidence rate of hospitalizations for asthma during long-term therapy was 92% lower in the omalizumab group than in the placebo group (omalizumab, 0.26/100 patient years; placebo, 3.42/100 patient years; $P < 0.002$). The rate of unscheduled, asthma-related outpatient visits was lower for the omalizumab-treated patients than for the placebo-treated patients (rate ratio, 0.60; $P < 0.01$), as was the rate of asthma-related emergency room visits (rate ratio, 0.47; $P = 0.05$).

In addition to monitoring exacerbation rates and corticosteroid use, asthma control can be assessed by assessing changes in the patient's quality of life. Several studies have used the well-established and validated Asthma Quality of Life Questionnaire (AQLQ) to evaluate the effect of omalizumab on patient quality of life. For example, Finn and colleagues analyzed data from 535 adults with severe asthma who received omalizumab or placebo for 52 weeks in a randomized, double-blind trial. The AQLQ was administered at baseline and at weeks 16, 28, and 52. At each time point, omalizumab-treated patients demonstrated statistically

13

significant improvements across all AQLQ domains, as well as in overall score. Moreover, a greater proportion of patients receiving omalizumab achieved a clinically meaningful improvement in asthma-related quality of life during each phase of the study. In addition, >50% of both patients and investigators rated treatment with omalizumab similarly as excellent or good compared with <40% of placebo recipients (**Figure 13.2**).

Safety of Omalizumab

More than 4000 patients have received omalizumab in placebo-controlled clinical trials and no serious adverse events have been consistently reported.

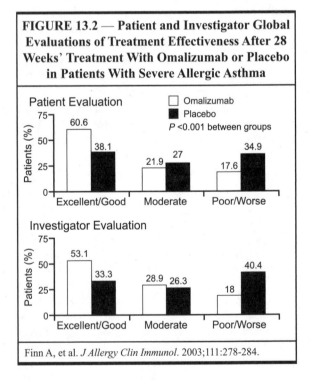

FIGURE 13.2 — Patient and Investigator Global Evaluations of Treatment Effectiveness After 28 Weeks' Treatment With Omalizumab or Placebo in Patients With Severe Allergic Asthma

Finn A, et al. *J Allergy Clin Immunol.* 2003;111:278-284.

Overall, the adverse events reported for patients treated with omalizumab compared with placebo have been similar and categorized as mild to moderate in severity. The most frequently reported adverse events were injection site reactions, fatigue, arthralgias, dizziness, itching, and dermatitis. In clinical trials to date, there has been no evidence or anti-IgE–IgE immune complex disease, nor has there been evidence of complement activation or fixation.

The prescribing information for omalizumab contains a warning regarding a possible increased risk of malignancy. Malignant neoplasms were observed in 20 (0.5%) of 4127 omalizumab-treated patients compared with five (0.2%) of 2236 control patients. The observed malignancies were of various types, including breast, nonmelanoma skin, melanoma, prostate, and parotid. Further postmarketing surveillance in progress will provide more definitive data on whether a causal relationship exists between malignancy and omalizumab.

Anaphylaxis occurred within 2 hours of the first or subsequent administration of omalizumab in three patients (<0.1%) without other identifiable allergic triggers. None of these patients required admission to an intensive care unit. Therefore, it is recommended that patients be observed after omalizumab injection, with medications immediately available for treatment of severe hypersensitivity reactions, including anaphylaxis.

Dosing of Omalizumab

Omalizumab is administered subcutaneously every 2 or 4 weeks at doses based on the patient's baseline serum IgE level and body weight. The monthly dose of omalizumab (in milligrams) is calculated as 0.016 mg × body weight in kg × the serum IgE level in IU/mL. Thus a 67-kg patient with an IgE level of 700 IU/mL would require 750 mg/month. However, owing to the volume of the injection, doses of omalizumab

>300 mg/month must be given in divided doses every 2 weeks (**Table 13.2**). Even so, some patients who are very large or have very high IgE levels, or both, may not be able to receive omalizumab because the calculated dose would still be too large to be given even in two injections per month. For example, a 65- kg patient with a serum IgE of 650 IU or a 95-kg patient with an IgE of 350 IU should not receive omalizumab.

Note also that administration of omalizumab is not recommended in patients in whom serum IgE level is <30 IU/mL because there is too little substrate for the omalizumab to bind.

Current Clinical Role of Omalizumab

Omalizumab represents a novel and efficacious form of therapy for patients with allergic asthma when used in the appropriate clinical setting. As discussed above, numerous clinical trials have demonstrated significant benefits in terms of reducing exacerbations in patients with moderate-to-severe persistent asthma. In addition, adding omalizumab to ICSs can result in significant reductions in the doses of steroids. Furthermore, omalizumab appears to be safe and well tolerated and may improve patient quality of life.

Omalizumab is not a first-line therapy for asthma and should not be used to treat acute exacerbations since it has no known benefit in such situations. It is intended for use only in patients who, despite optimal medications taken regularly, do not achieve the goals of asthma management. Therefore, it will usually be used as add-on therapy for patients already using ICS preparations, and perhaps one or more other drugs such as long-acting β-agonists.

The Food and Drug Administration has approved omalizumab for use in patients who meet all of the following criteria:

- Moderate or severe persistent allergic asthma

TABLE 13.2 — Omalizumab Doses (mg) Administered Subcutaneously Every 4 Weeks or Every 2 Weeks (Shaded Blocks)

Pretreatment Serum IgE (IU/mL)	Body Weight (kg)			
	30-60	>60-70	>70-90	>90-150
30-100	150	150	150	300
>100-200	300	300	300	225
>200-300	300	225	225	300
>300-400	225	225	300	Do not dose
>400-500	300	300	375	Do not dose
>500-600	300	375	Do not dose	Do not dose
>600-700	375	Do not dose	Do not dose	Do not dose

13

- Age >12 years
- A pretreatment serum IgE level between 30 and 700 IU/mL
- A positive result on skin-prick testing or radioallerogosorbent testing with at least one perennial allergen.

Since biologic agents, such as omalizumab, tend to be expensive to produce and administer, cost-effectiveness is of some concern when considering the appropriate and optimal use of omalizumab. Given that patients with severe asthma incur considerable annual costs for medications, emergency department treatments, and hospitalizations, perhaps as high as $12,800 per year, the demonstrated ability of omalizumab to reduce the rates of exacerbations, emergency department visits, and hospitalizations suggests that it likely would be cost-effective in many patients with poorly controlled allergic asthma. Several studies have in fact shown omalizumab to be cost-effective when used in the type of patients for which it is currently indicated. Unlike most other biologic agents, the monthly dose of omalizumab, and hence its cost, will vary from patient to patient. For example, a 300-mg/month dose for a 50-kg patient with a 300 IU/mL IgE level would cost about half that for the 600-mg monthly dose required for an 85-kg patient with a 400 IU/mL IgE level. Thus the cost-effectiveness of omalizumab should be assessed in terms of a patient's clinical needs and the cost of the appropriate omalizumab dose.

SUGGESTED READING

Ayres JG, Higgins B, Chilvers ER, Ayre G, Blogg M, Fox H. Efficacy and tolerability of anti-immunoglobulin E therapy with omalizumab in patients with poorly controlled (moderate-to-severe) allergic asthma. *Allergy*. 2004;59:701-708.

Buhl R, Hanf G, Soler M, et al. The anti-IgE antibody omalizumab improves asthma-related quality of life in patients with allergic asthma. *Eur Respir J*. 2002;20:1088-1094.

Burrows B, Martinez FD, Halonen M, Barbee RA, Cline MG. Association of asthma with serum IgE levels and skin-test reactivity to allergens. *N Engl J Med*. 1989;320:271-277.

Busse W, Corren J, Lanier BQ, et al. Omalizumab, anti-IgE recombinant humanized monoclonal antibody, for the treatment of severe allergic asthma. *J Allergy Clin Immunol*. 2001;108:184-190.

Chiang DT, Clark J, Casale TB. Omalizumab in asthma: approval and postapproval experience. *Clin Rev Allergy Immunol*. 2005;29:3-16.

Corren J, Casale T, Deniz Y, Ashby M. Omalizumab, a recombinant humanized anti-IgE antibody, reduces asthma-related emergency room visits and hospitalizations in patients with allergic asthma. *J Allergy Clin Immunol*. 2003;111:87-90.

D'Amato G. Role of anti-IgE monoclonal antibody (omalizumab) in the treatment of bronchial asthma and allergic respiratory diseases. *Eur J Pharmacol*. 2006;533:302-307.

Fahy JV, Fleming HE, Wong HH, et al. The effect of an anti-IgE monoclonal antibody on the early- and late-phase responses to allergen inhalation in asthmatic subjects. *Am J Respir Crit Care Med*. 1997;155:1828-1834.

Finn A, Gross G, van Bavel J, et al. Omalizumab improves asthma-related quality of life in patients with severe allergic asthma. *J Allergy Clin Immunol*. 2003;111:278-284.

Holgate S, Bousquet J, Wenzel S, Fox H, Liu J, Castellsague J. Efficacy of omalizumab, an anti-immunoglobulin E antibody, in patients with allergic asthma at high risk of serious asthma-related morbidity and mortality. *Curr Med Res Opin*. 2001;17:233-240.

Holgate S, Casale T, Wenzel S, Bousquet J, Deniz Y, Reisner C. The anti-inflammatory effects of omalizumab confirm the central role of IgE in allergic inflammation. *J Allergy Clin Immunol*. 2005;115:459-465.

Holgate ST, Chuchalin AG, Hebert J, et al. Efficacy and safety of a recombinant anti-immunoglobulin E antibody (omalizumab) in severe allergic asthma. *Clin Exp Allergy*. 2004;34:632-638.

13

Lanier BQ, Corren J, Lumry W, Liu J, Fowler-Taylor A, Gupta N. Omalizumab is effective in the long-term control of severe allergic asthma. *Ann Allergy Asthma Immunol.* 2003;91:154-159.

Lemanske RF Jr, Nayak A, McAlary M, Everhard F, Fowler-Taylor A, Gupta N. Omalizumab improves asthma-related quality of life in children with allergic asthma. *Pediatrics.* 2002;110:e55.

Luskin AT, Kosinski M, Bresnahan BW, Ashby M, Wong DA. Symptom control and improved functioning: the effect of omalizumab on asthma-related quality of life (ARQL). *J Asthma.* 2005;42:823-827.

MacGlashan DW Jr, Bochner BS, Adelman DC, et al. Down-regulation of Fc (epsilon) RI expression on human basophils during in vivo treatment of atopic patients with anti-IgE antibody. *J Immunol.* 1997;158:1438-1445.

Milgrom H, Berger W, Nayak A, et al. Treatment of childhood asthma with anti-immunoglobulin E antibody (omalizumab). *Pediatrics.* 2001;108:E36.

Oba Y, Salzman GA. Cost-effectiveness analysis of omalizumab in adults and adolescents with moderate-to-severe allergic asthma. *J Allergy Clin Immunol.* 2004;114:265-269.

Poole JA, Matangkasombut P, Rosenwasser LJ. Targeting the IgE molecule in allergic and asthmatic diseases: review of the IgE molecule and clinical efficacy. *J Allergy Clin Immunol.* 2005;115(suppl):S376-S385.

Rambasek TE, Lang DM, Kavuru MS. Omalizumab: where does it fit into current asthma management? *Cleve Clin J Med.* 2004;71:251-61.

Sears MR, Burrows B, Flannery EM, Herbison GP, Hewitt CJ, Holdaway MD. Relation between airway responsiveness and serum IgE in children with asthma and in apparently normal children. *N Engl J Med.* 1991;325:1067-1071.

Soler M, Matz J, Townley R, et al. The anti-IgE antibody omalizumab reduces exacerbations and steroid requirement in allergic asthmatics. *Eur Respir J.* 2001;18:254-261.

Sunyer J, Anto JM, Sabria J, et al. Relationship between serum IgE and airway responsiveness in adults with asthma. *J Allergy Clin Immunol.* 1995;95:699-706.

14 Alternative Therapies

A minority of asthma patients—perhaps 5% to 10%—continue to have troublesome symptoms with frequent exacerbations that necessitate hospitalization despite maximal conventional therapy. The reversible factors that contribute to steroid-dependent asthma include:

- Noncompliance
- Poor self-management strategies
- Inadequate control of allergen burden at home
- Inadequate inhaler technique
- Suboptimal pharmacotherapy.

The placebo arm of a number of studies has clearly shown that a compulsive traditional management plan, with frequent follow-up (perhaps in an asthma center), can reduce the need for oral steroids by 16% to 40% in steroid-dependent asthma. Numerous studies have demonstrated the efficacy of alternative anti-inflammatory therapies that provide a steroid-sparing effect in asthma. Methotrexate, gold salts, troleandomycin (TAO), cyclosporine, colchicine, chloroquine, gamma globulin, and dapsone are some of the agents that have been investigated.

Glucocorticoid-Resistant Asthma

Carmichael and colleagues described 58 patients with chronic asthma in whom the forced expiratory volume in 1 second (FEV_1) increased <15% after a 7-day course of at least 20 mg prednisolone daily. Dykewicz and colleagues studied the natural history of asthma in 40 randomly selected adults with asthma refractory to inhaled beclomethasone and β-agonists and dependent on long-term prednisone therapy (mean duration 6.2 ± 5 years). Over 3 to 5 years, 24 patients (60%) had unchanged prednisone requirements, 13 patients (32.5%) improved and required less prednisone, and three patients (7.5%) deteriorated and required more prednisone. Unfortunately, this study did not report the maintenance dose of beclomethasone.

Corrigan and coworkers evaluated the possible mechanism of chronic asthma in patients with clinical glucocorticoid resistance (<30% increase in FEV_1 after 2 weeks of daily prednisone treatment, 20 mg for the first week and 40 mg for the second week). Glucocorticoid pharmacokinetics, receptor characteristics, and inhibition of peripheral blood T-cell proliferation by prednisone were assayed. Overall, the investigators noted a relative insensitivity of T lymphocytes to prednisone in patients with clinical glucocorticoid resistance compared with matched glucocorticoid-sensitive patients. They noted that resistance does not reflect abnormal glucocorticoid clearance. Additional studies by this group suggested that activated T lymphocytes may be the target, and perhaps an anti–T lymphocyte drug, such as cyclosporine, may be particularly useful in glucocorticoid-resistant asthma. Overall, the clinical relevance of glucocorticoid resistance in patients with chronic steroid-dependent asthma remains speculative and poorly understood.

Methotrexate

Methotrexate, an inhibitor of dihydrofolate reductase, appears to inhibit neutrophil-dependent inflammation. Methotrexate has been evaluated in steroid-dependent asthma in eleven controlled clinical trials between 1988 and 1996, following long experience with this drug in rheumatoid arthritis and psoriasis.

Mullarkey and associates conducted a placebo-controlled, crossover study in 14 steroid-dependent asthma patients. The average dose was 26 mg/day (range 10 mg to 60 mg). Patients were randomly assigned to receive either placebo or methotrexate (15 mg by mouth per week) for 12 weeks, and then were switched to the alternate form of therapy. They were seen every 3 weeks in follow-up. On the average, patients needed 36.5% less prednisone when they were receiving methotrexate than when they received placebo.

The same group published a follow-up experience of 31 cushingoid asthma patients who were receiving prednisone and inhaled corticosteroids daily. Patients were treated with low-dose methotrexate for 18 to 28 months. The mean prednisone dose declined from 26.9 mg/day to 6.2 mg/day in the 25 patients who completed the study, and 15 patients stopped using prednisone regularly.

Similarly, Shiner and coworkers conducted a 24-week, placebo-controlled trial in 69 steroid-dependent asthma patients. The mean daily prednisolone dose was 14.2 mg/day. During 12 weeks of treatment, steroid doses were tapered by 16% in both the methotrexate and placebo groups. However, between 12 and 24 weeks, the prednisolone dose was reduced more in the methotrexate group than in the placebo group (50% vs 14%). Patients were evaluated every 4 weeks in the study. Five of the 38 patients taking methotrexate had liver function abnormalities.

14

Erzurum and colleagues conducted a double-blind, parallel-group study over 13 weeks of prednisone-dependent asthma (average daily dose 20 mg, range 15 mg to 30 mg), in which 19 patients received either methotrexate (15 mg intramuscularly every week) or placebo. This study was unique in that patients were seen weekly and there was a 1-month baseline period during which conventional therapy was maximized and attempts to reduce the baseline prednisone dose were made. Overall, both groups reduced their oral prednisone dose by about 40%. The authors concluded that methotrexate did not produce significant benefit in corticosteroid-dependent asthma.

More recently, a meta-analysis attempted to combine the results of 11 published trials of methotrexate for steroid-dependent asthma. Overall, six of 11 studies concluded that methotrexate did not have a steroid-sparing effect. The average steroid dose at initiation of these studies was 18.4 mg/d and methotrexate treatment decreased steroid usage by 4.37 mg/day or 23.7% of initial dosage ($P < 0.05$). Subgroup analysis showed greatest steroid-sparing effects with:

- Methotrexate therapy ≥ 6 months
- Low, long-term steroid therapy (≤ 20 mg/d)
- Study design incorporating a run-in period.

In summary, based on the available studies, it is difficult to recommend therapy with methotrexate outside the setting of a clinical trial..

Gold

Both oral and parenteral gold preparations have been used in studies of steroid-dependent asthma. In general, the addition of gold decreased corticosteroid requirements, improved symptoms, and perhaps improved bronchial hyperreactivity as well. However, these studies had a number of methodologic limitations. Further, overall patient tolerance was poor: the incidence of side effects, including diarrhea, skin eruptions, and proteinuria was as high as 37%.

A recent 8-month controlled trial of 227 steroid-dependent asthmatics (prednisone ≥ 10 mg/d) randomized patients to oral gold (auranofin 4 mg twice daily) or placebo. Significant reduction in oral steroid dose ($\geq 50\%$ of baseline) was achieved in the auranofin group (60%) compared with the placebo group (32%) (P <0.001). Gastrointestinal and cutaneous adverse effects were greater in the auranofin group.

Troleandomycin

Another steroid-sparing approach in the treatment of chronic asthma is the use of TAO, a macrolide antibiotic. A number of open-label studies have demonstrated a reduction in corticosteroid dose when this drug was added to the regimen. The principal effect of TAO is the prolongation of the plasma half-life of corticosteroids through the inhibition of their elimination; in one study, the methylprednisolone half-life increased from 2.46 hours before TAO therapy to 4.63 hours 1 week after TAO therapy. Published protocols highlight the importance of using methylprednisolone rather than prednisone in conjunction with TAO to have the steroid-sparing effect.

A recent, 2-year, placebo-controlled, parallel-group study was performed in 75 steroid-dependent asthma patients to compare TAO plus methylprednisolone vs methylprednisolone alone. Patents in both groups achieved alternate-day steroid therapy and the reduction in methylprednisolone dose was not significantly different between the treatment groups. However, the patients in the TAO group had significantly more steroid-related side effects as assessed by serum levels of immunoglobulin G (IgG), glucose, and cholesterol, and as reflected by osteoporosis. This well-designed study strongly supports the notion that the steroid-sparing properties of TAO are a pharmacologic phenomenon that does not translate into fewer long-term steroid-related side effects. This study indicated that further trials with TAO are probably not indicated.

14

Cyclosporine

The immunosuppressive agent cyclosporin A (CsA) inhibits mediator release from mast cells and basophils and inhibits the syntheses of lymphokines, with the subsequent down-regulation of CD_4^+ T lymphocytes playing a critical role in chronic asthma. A number of investigators have evaluated cyclosporine in steroid-dependent asthma. Alexander and associates conducted a double-blind, placebo-controlled, crossover trial of cyclosporine (initial 2-week washout period). In 30 of 33 patients in the cyclosporine group, the peak expiratory flow rate and FEV_1 increased significantly and the frequency of disease exacerbations was 48% lower. Corticosteroid dosage reduction was not attempted in this study.

More recently, Lock and associates conducted a 36-week, placebo-controlled, randomized, double-blind trial using CsA (5 mg/kg/d) in 39 steroid-dependent asthmatic patients. The 16/19 patients who completed CsA therapy achieved a significant reduction in prednisone dosage of 62% (10 mg to 3.5 mg) compared with 25% (10 mg to 7.5 mg) in the placebo group ($P = 0.04$). Side effects occurred more often in the CsA group, but these did not require withdrawal from the study. The well-known side effects of CsA include:

- Hypertension
- Hypertrichosis
- Neurologic disturbances
- Nephrotoxicity.

Overall, no alternative anti-inflammatory agent has been proven to be superior to steroids in the treatment of asthma, and the use of such therapies should be restricted to clinical trials only.

SUGGESTED READING

Alexander AG, Barnes NC, Kay AB. Trial of cyclosporin in corticosteroid-dependent chronic severe asthma. *Lancet.* 1992;339:324-328.

Barnes PJ. Immunomodulation as asthma therapy: where do we stand? *Eur Respir J.* 1996;22(suppl):154s-159s.

Barnes PJ. New drugs for asthma. *Eur Respir J.* 1992;5:1126-1136.

Bernstein IL, Bernstein DI, Dubb JW, Faiferman I, Wallin B. A placebo-controlled multicenter study of auranofin in the treatment of patients with corticosteriod-dependent asthma. Auranofin Multicenter Drug Trial. *J Allergy Clin Immunol.* 1996;98:317-324.

Carmichael J, Paterson IC, Diaz P, Crompton GK, Kay AB, Grant IW. Corticosteroid resistance in chronic asthma. *Br Med J.* 1981; 282:1419-1422.

Coffey MJ, Sanders G, Eschenbacher WL, et al. The role of methotrexate in the management of steroid-dependent asthma. *Chest.* 1994;105:117-121.

Corrigan CJ, Brown PH, Barnes NC, et al. Glucocorticoid resistance in chronic asthma. *Am Rev Respir Dis.* 1991;144(suppl):1016-1032.

Dykewicz MS, Greenberger PA, Patterson R, Halwig JM. Natural history of asthma in patients requiring long-term systemic corticosteroids. *Arch Intern Med.* 1986;146:2369-2372.

Erzurum SC, Leff JA, Cochran JE, et al. Lack of benefit of methotrexate in severe steroid-dependent asthma. *Ann Intern Med.* 1991; 114:353-360.

Lane DJ, Lane TV. Alternative and complementary medicine for asthma. *Thorax.* 1991;46:787-797.

Lock SH, Kay AB, Barnes NC. Double-blind, placebo-controlled study of cyclosporin A as a corticosteroid-sparing agent in corticosteroid-dependent asthma. *Am J Respir Crit Care Med.* 1996; 153:509-514.

Marin MG. Low-dose methotrexate spares steroid usage in steroid-dependent asthmatic patients: a meta-analysis. *Chest.* 1997;112:29-33.

14

Mullarkey MF, Lammert JK, Blumenstein BA. Long-term methotrexate treatment in corticosteroid-dependent asthma. *Ann Intern
Med.* 1990;112:577-581.

Nelson HS, Hamilos DL, Corsello PR, Levesque NV, Buchmeier AD,
Bucher BL. A double-blind study of troleandomycin and methylpred-
nisolone in asthmatic subjects who require daily corticosteroids. *Am
Rev Respir Dis.* 1993;147:398-404.

Newman KB, Mason UG, Buchmeier A, Schmaling KB, Corsello
P, Nelson HS. Failure of colchicine to reduce inhaled triamcinolone
dose in patients with asthma. *J Allergy Clin Immunol.* 1997;99:176-
178.

Shiner RJ, Nunn AJ, Chung KF, Geddes DM. Randomised, double-
blind, placebo-controlled trial of methotrexate in steroid-dependent
asthma. *Lancet.* 1990;336:137-140.

15   Status Asthmaticus

Introduction

Status asthmaticus is an acute, severe exacerbation of asthma that requires care in a hospital setting. Recent epidemiologic data for acute asthma suggest there are about 500,000 hospitalizations for this condition per year in the United States, of which 65% occur in patients >18 years of age. Acute asthma represents 4% of all emergency department (ED) visits involving about 2 million people. Between 15% and 25% of the ED visits for acute asthma result in hospital admission. About 20% to 30% of patients initially managed and discharged from the ED experience a relapse. The average length of stay for patients admitted to the hospital is about 5 days. Of all hospital admissions, about 4% require intensive care and of these, 1% to 30% require mechanical ventilation.

Patients typically come to the ED and/or hospital for acute asthma when the episode is severe and the tempo of illness is progressive and/or unresponsive to initial therapy. Acute asthma exacerbation often represents failure of outpatient maintenance therapy for several possible reasons:

- Lack of access to longitudinal medical care
- Lack of objective monitoring of asthma, including home peak-flow monitoring
- Poor self-management skills
- Inadequate pharmacotherapy prescription by the physician (most often lack of inhaled corticosteroid maintenance therapy).

For some patients, acute asthma exacerbation may be complicated by a comorbid illness that makes outpatient management difficult, such as psychiatric illness. Of course, a subset of patients use the ED as the point of access for longitudinal subacute care. The clinician caring for the patient with status asthmaticus in either the ED or hospital setting faces several questions:

- What is the best initial therapy?
- What clinical or physiologic parameters determine success or failure?
- What are the criteria for admission to the floor vs the intensive care unit?
- If the initial therapy fails, what are the issues related to mechanical ventilation and "salvage therapy"?

This chapter will consider some of these issues.

Management

■ Bronchodilators

The initial management of an acute asthmatic in any setting should include administration of aerosolized β-agonists on a repeated basis. See **Figure 7.1** and **Figure 7.2** for an overview of therapy for acute asthma, recommended by the 2007 National Asthma Education and Prevention Program (NAEPP) guidelines. β-Agonists may be administered by:

- Metered-dose inhaler (MDI) with a spacer device
- Intermittent bolus nebulization
- Continuous nebulization.

Comparable clinical effects can be achieved with all three delivery methods. Evidence suggests that patients with acute, severe airflow obstruction need higher doses of aerosolized β-agonists than patients with less severe stable airflow obstruction. Selective β_2-agonists such as albuterol (2.5 mg/dose) or metaproterenol (15 mg/dose) are preferred over isoetharine (5 mg/dose).

The potency ratio of a nebulizer to an MDI with spacer device is 7:1; therefore, one nebulization with 2.5 mg albuterol is roughly equivalent to 4 to 12 puffs of an albuterol MDI delivering 90 mcg/puff (the equivalent dose range for the MDI is 0.36 to 1.08 mg). In a normal person, only 10% of the MDI dose reaches the lower airway; whereas in patients with airflow obstruction, about 6% reaches the lower airway with 3% to the distal-most airways. Use of a spacer device roughly doubles this amount.

A number of studies have suggested that β-agonists may be effective and safe when given continuously by a variety of nebulization devices for up to 72 or 96 hours in children. Two recent studies have extended these findings to adults as well. Patients with acute airflow obstruction refractory to intermittent, frequent, aerosolized β-agonist therapy may be candidates for continuous therapy with a nebulized bronchodilator while awaiting the effects of anti-inflammatory therapy. Recommended dosages are:

- Albuterol 2.5 mg to 15 mg/hour
- Terbutaline 2 mg to 8 mg/hour.

Extensive experience in children and the two studies in adults suggest that this approach is safe, although further studies in adults with underlying coronary artery disease are required. It is important to remember that patients who are undergoing this therapy should be monitored closely.

Over the past 10 years, there has been a strong shift away from the use of parenteral β-agonist therapy in adults. There is essentially no role for intravenous β-agonists in the care of acute asthmatics. Aerosolized β-agonists are the preferred bronchodilator for initial therapy for acute asthma due to their:

- Rapid onset
- Superior bronchodilation.

However, anticholinergic agents have also been used. A review of recently published trials suggests that β-agonists are superior to anticholinergics and that the combination of β-aerosols with anticholinergics is modestly better (10% to 20%) than the use of β-agonists alone. It may be reasonable to use aerosolized ipratropium in addition to β-agonists in patients with severe acute asthma.

The role of methylxanthines in the acute management of asthma is limited. Theophylline is inferior to an inhaled β-agonist as a bronchodilator. Also, the addition of theophylline to maximal therapy with β-aerosols and systemic corticosteroids does not appear to confer a benefit in the first 4 to 6 hours. A large meta-analysis of 13 published studies does not support the use of theophylline. The EPR-2 does not recommend methylxanthines for acute asthma. If a patient is on maintenance therapy with theophylline, therapy can be continued orally or, if the drug level is low, by bolus and intravenous (IV) infusion.

■ Corticosteroids

Systemic corticosteroids should be administered to most patients with acute asthma exacerbation in an ED setting. Data suggest that early use of these agents will:

- Lessen the need for hospital admission
- Reduce the relapse rate for discharged patients
- Shorten the length of stay in the hospital for those admitted.

The onset of beneficial effects of systemic steroids will take a minimum of 4 to 8 hours. Much has been written about the dose of systemic corticosteroids, but it is general practice to use methylprednisolone intravenously 60 mg to 125 mg every 6 to 8 hours or prednisone 30 mg to 60 mg orally every 6 hours. Data clearly suggest these doses are effective and well tolerated, but the minimum required doses are not very well established.

Fanta and associates demonstrated that in patients with acute severe episodes of asthma refractory to 8 hours of conventional bronchodilator therapy, the subjects given intravenous corticosteroids had significantly greater resolution of airflow obstruction by the end of 24 hours. Littenberg demonstrated that prompt use of glucocorticoids in the emergency treatment of severe asthma can:

- Prevent significant morbidity
- Reduce the number of hospitalizations
- Affect substantial savings in health care costs.

Other studies have shown that the use of oral steroids can decrease the need for hospitalization for patients presenting to the ED with acute asthma exacerbation. Oral steroids are well absorbed from the gastrointestinal tract; therefore, oral therapy represents a reasonable, cost-effective alternative to the conventional IV therapy. The optimal schedule for steroid tapering following an acute exacerbation is not well established. In one study, Lederle and colleagues suggested that the relapse rate was not different between a steroid taper over 2 weeks compared with 8 weeks, although the relapse rate was quite high in both groups.

Therefore, the conventional therapy for acute severe asthma exacerbation would include:

- Oxygen
- Repeated aerosolized β-agonists
- Systemic corticosteroids.

Forced hydration and antibiotics are usually not required. Reassessment at frequent intervals by physical examination and peak-flow meter should be performed to determine whether the patient is improving, staying about the same, or deteriorating. Response to therapy is probably the single most important factor in helping to determine the need for hospital admission. Some commonly used criteria are listed in **Table 15.1**. It is true that patients showing improvement on this therapy and discharged home with oral corticosteroids do well without significant relapse. A practical duration of treatment in a typical ED setting is about 4 hours. If a patient requires further therapy after 4 hours, the next decision is whether to admit the patient for prolonged inpatient care or continue therapy in the setting of an ED-based observation unit or holding room when these facilities are available. There are conflicting data on whether these observation units (typically consisting of care for 12 to 24 hours):

- Lessen the need for hospital admission
- Reduce the total length of stay
- Are cost-effective.

For patients who are admitted to the hospital, the next decision is whether to manage them on a regular nursing floor or in the intensive-care unit (ICU). Patients with severe airflow obstruction who are deteriorating despite conventional therapy (based on evidence of respiratory muscle fatigue and/or respiratory depression) should be managed in a closely monitored intensive-care setting to serially assess the need for airway support and mechanical ventilation. This may be initiated in the ED. For all other patients, therapy could be continued on a regular floor with frequent "q-2-hour" administration of aerosolized β-agonists and serial peak-flow measurement.

■ Unconventional Therapies

Most patients with acute asthma respond to aggressive conventional therapy with aerosolized β-agonists and systemic corticosteroids. However, for the subset of patients with delayed or inadequate response to

TABLE 15.1 — Proposed Spirometric Criteria for Hospital Admission

Basis	Indications for Admission
Initial presentation	• Fischl index ≥ 4* • Inability to perform spirometry • FEV_1 <0.61 L
Initial flow rate and response to first treatment	• Unresponsive to epinephrine and PEF <60 L/min • Unresponsive to bronchodilators and <16% change in initial PEF value • <0.15 L increase in FEV_1 after subcutaneous administration of bronchodilator • PEF <100 L/min initially and <160 L/min after 0.25 mg terbutaline • FEV_1 <30% of predicted value; not improving to >40% of predicted value; >4 hours therapy needed
Initial flow rate and response to full treatment	• PEF <100 L/min and <300 L/min after full treatment • FEV_1 <0.61 L and <1.6 L after full treatment • Change in FEV_1 <0.4 L after bronchodilator administration • Deterioration of PEF by 15% after initial good response to bronchodilator therapy

Abbreviations: FEV_1, forced expiratory volume in 1 second; PEF, peak expiratory flow.

* See *Identifying High-Risk Patients and Hospital Admission Criteria* in Chapter 5, *Clinical Evaluation and Assessment of Severity*.

Modified from: Brenner BE. *Am J Emerg Med.* 1985;3:74-77.

15

initial therapy, a variety of unconventional therapies may be considered. These include the use of:

- IV magnesium
- Mixture of helium-oxygen gas
- Noninvasive ventilation
- Ketamine
- Inhalational anesthetics.

There are published reports in support of each of these therapies. However, these therapies should be considered experimental and be reserved for patients who are not improving despite maximal conventional therapy. The rationale for the use of IV magnesium is based on the fact that magnesium:

- Inhibits calcium channels
- Reduces the acetylcholine release
- May improve respiratory muscle function.

In addition, the serum level of magnesium may be low in 50% of patients with acute asthma exacerbation. Although there are a number of uncontrolled studies which have shown beneficial effects with IV magnesium, at least two randomized clinical trials have not.

Heliox is a blend of helium and oxygen; when inhaled by an asthmatic, turbulent flow in narrowed airways may become laminar, thereby reducing the resistive work of breathing. Several prospective, uncontrolled studies, have shown improvement in:

- Peak flows
- Respiratory muscle fatigue
- Reversal of hypercapnia.

It is important to recognize that the Heliox mixture typically uses 60% to 80% helium; therefore, patients who are severely hypoxemic are not appropriate candidates.

Noninvasive, positive-pressure ventilation has been used for patients with acute asthma with inadequate initial response to therapy. Several uncontrolled small series and case reports suggest that continuous positive airway pressure therapy with 5 cm to 7.5 cm H_2O can help unload the inspiratory muscles and avoid intubation. The use of this modality is labor intensive and should be reserved for a small number of carefully selected patients in the ICU.

■ Mechanical Ventilation

A small subset of patients may have such severe airflow obstruction and airway inflammation so as not to be able to maintain spontaneous ventilation despite aggressive initial therapy. These patients require intubation and mechanical ventilation in an intensive-care setting.

The intubation itself may occur:
• In the field
• In an ED
• On a regular nursing floor
• In the ICU.

Technically, these patients are difficult to intubate because they are quite tachypneic and in respiratory distress, they do not tolerate lying flat, and their airways are hyperreactive.

Optimizing the conditions for intubation includes using the most experienced operator, intubating in a controlled elective setting, and by the appropriate use of sedating agents. Good sedating agents to facilitate intubation include:

15

• Midazolam (a short-acting benzodiazepine)
• Ketamine
• Propofol.

It is best to avoid morphine at the time of intubation since it can produce hypotension, induce nausea and emesis, and contribute to bronchospasm by histamine release. Ketamine, a phencyclidine that inhibits the reuptake of catecholamine, is commonly used as an induction agent prior to administration of a general anesthetic. It has a rapid onset, is short acting and has the advantages of being a bronchodilator, a vagolytic agent, and perhaps an anti-inflammatory agent. A typical dose is 0.1 mg/kg to 0.2 mg/kg IV bolus followed by 0.5 mg/kg delivered by infusion over a 3-hour period. Ketamine has the potential to increase heart rate and blood pressure and lower the seizure threshold. A recent, prospective, randomized trial compared the addition of ketamine to the therapy for acute asthmatics refractory to initial ED therapy with three doses of inhaled β-agonists and systemic steroids. Compared to placebo, ketamine did not show benefit.

Early studies of the use of mechanical ventilation in patients with status asthmaticus in the 1970s indicated significant mortality (9% to 38%) and significant iatrogenic complications. However, over the past 20 years, the prognosis for ventilated acute asthmatics seems to have improved dramatically. More recent studies show a low death rate and a relatively low complication rate. The key principle that has evolved for mechanical ventilation of patients with status asthmaticus is controlled hypoventilation. The goal of mechanical ventilation in these patients is to:

- Support oxygenation
- Have an acceptable pH
- Avoid iatrogenic complications related to increased intrathoracic pressures.

The complications of mechanical ventilation for status asthmaticus are due to incomplete emptying of the lungs, gas trapping, or auto-positive end-expiratory pressure (PEEP). Normalization of the partial pressure of carbon dioxide should not be a goal and "permissive hypercapnia" should be accepted with a pH of 7.2 to 7.3. Occasionally, supplementation with intravenous bicarbonate is required. The specific ventilatory

216

strategies to minimize airway pressure and auto-PEEP involve (**Table 15.2**):

- Reducing the minute ventilation by reducing the rate, tidal volume, or both with the ventilator as well as with adequate sedation
- Reducing the inspiratory time and increasing the expiratory time by increasing the inspiratory flow rate by which the tidal volume is delivered.

TABLE 15.2 — Strategies and Goals for Mechanical Ventilation in Status Asthmaticus

- Assure adequate oxygenation
- Minimize risk of barotrauma
  - Attempt to keep plateau pressure <30 cm to 40 cm H_2O
  - Tolerate hypercapnia with pH >7.20
- Use bicarbonate therapy if needed
- Minimize auto-PEEP
  - Reduce minute ventilation
  - Increase expiratory time by reducing the rate and increasing the flow rate
- Assure adequate sedation
- Avoid neuromuscular blocking agents

Abbreviation: PEEP, positive end-expiratory pressure.

The net effect of these changes is to lessen the risk of barotrauma and hypotension. Patients who are being mechanically ventilated by this strategy will require heavy sedation with benzodiazepines or propofol, and every effort should be made to avoid neuromuscular blockade. Patients with status asthmaticus are typically treated with systemic corticosteroids, and the combination of steroid and neuromuscular blockers seems to be a significant risk factor for the catastrophic development of prolonged paralysis. Although the exact mechanism for this phenomenon is unknown, it is thought to be either a myopathic and/or neuropathic injury. Therefore, neuromuscular blockade should be

15

reserved for patients who otherwise could not be supported by a mechanical ventilator.

While patients are being treated with nebulized β-agonists and systemic corticosteroids and supported with mechanical ventilation, a number of heroic salvage therapies have been performed with anecdotal success. These include the use of inhalational anesthetics and bronchoalveolar lavage. Anesthetic agents are thought to be effective because they potentiate β_2-receptors and they have direct bronchodilator properties. Anesthetics are effective even in the presence of acidosis. However, these agents (including halothane and ether) have adverse effects, including myocardial depression and irritability, along with idiosyncratic reactions. More importantly, these agents are typically not familiar to medical ICU personnel and present various logistics for use. Inhalational anesthetics should be reserved for the rarest situation where there is expertise in the use of these agents in the intensive-care setting. Limited data suggest that alveolar lavage, with either saline or acetylcysteine, may remove mucous plugs and improve airflow and oxygenation.

■ Summary

Asthma should be viewed largely as an outpatient disease. It is likely that outcomes for chronic asthma will be improved by:
- Aggressive patient education in self-management skills
- Objective monitoring of early exacerbations
- Wide use of anti-inflammatory therapy.

However, for a variety of reasons, a subset of patients will not have access to this therapy or this therapy will fail resulting in life-threatening episodes of acute asthma. Aggressive therapy for status asthmaticus involves repeated aerosolized bronchodilators and systemic corticosteroids. This should be performed in a setting of frequent objective monitoring of peak flows and/or blood gases. The vast majority of patients will improve. Patients who are refractory to this therapy should be observed in a hospital/ICU setting for more gradual improvement. Mechanical ventilation in patients with status asthmaticus requires special ventilator strategies to minimize iatrogenic complications. Ultimately, the primary goal of hospitalization in such patients is to equip them with skills, tools, and medications to avoid future episodes of acute exacerbation. It is true that a history of prior hospitalization and/or respiratory failure is a significant predictor of poor outcome, including mortality, which should be considered preventable.

SUGGESTED READING

Aelony Y. "Noninvasive" oral treatment of asthma in the emergency room. *Am J Med.* 1985;78:929-936.

Braman SS, Kaemmerlen JT. Intensive care of status asthmaticus. A 10-year experience. *JAMA.* 1990;264:366-368.

Brenner BE. The acute asthmatic in the emergency department: the decision to admit or discharge. *Am J Emerg Med.* 1985;3:74-77.

Clinical Practice Guidelines. Expert Panel Report 2: Guidelines for the Diagnosis and Management of Asthma. Bethesda, Md: US Dept of Health and Human Services; 1997. NIH publication 97-4051.

Corbridge TC, Hall JB. The assessment and management of adults with status asthmaticus. *Am J Respir Crit Care Med.* 1995;151: 1296-1316.

Fanta CH, Rossing TH, McFadden ER Jr. Glucocorticoids in acute asthma. A critical controlled trial. *Am J Med.* 1983;74:845-851.

Howton JC, Rose J, Duffy S, Zoltanski T, Levitt MA. Randomized, double-blind, placebo-controlled trial of intravenous ketamine in acute asthma. *Ann Emerg Med.* 1996;27:170-175.

Kavuru MS. Beta-agonists for acute asthma: which way to deliver? *J Respir Dis.* 1994;15:312-314.

15

Kelly HW, Murphy S. Should anticholinergics be used in acute severe asthma? *DICP*. 1990;24:409-416.

Lederle FA, Pluhar RE, Joseph AM, Niewoehner DE. Tapering of corticosteroid therapy following exacerbation of asthma. A randomized, double-blind, placebo-controlled trial. *Arch Intern Med*. 1987; 147:2201-2203.

Littenberg B. Aminophylline in severe, acute asthma. A meta-analysis. *JAMA*. 1988;259:1678-1684.

Manthous CA. Management of severe exacerbations of asthma. *Am J Med*. 1995;99:298-308.

Marquette CH, Saulnier F, Leroy O, et al. Long-term prognosis of near-fatal asthma. A 6-year follow-up study of 145 asthmatic patients who underwent mechanical ventilation for a near-fatal attack of asthma. *Am Rev Respir Dis*. 1992;146:76-81.

Mayo PH, Richman J, Harris HW. Results of a program to reduce admissions for adult asthma. *Ann Intern Med*. 1990;112:864-871.

McFadden ER Jr. Dosages of corticosteroids in asthma. *Am Rev Respir Dis*. 1993;147:1306-1310.

McFadden ER Jr, Elsanadi N, Dixon L, et al. Protocol therapy for acute asthma: therapeutic benefits and cost savings. *Am J Med*. 1995;99:651-661.

McFadden ER Jr, Elsanadi N, Strauss L, et al. The influence of parasympatholytics on the resolution of acute attacks of asthma. *Am J Med*. 1997;102:7-13.

Reed CE, Hunt LW. The emergency visit and management of asthma. *Ann Intern Med*. 1990;112:801-802. Editorial.

Rossing TH, Fanta CH, Goldstein DH, Snapper JR, McFadden ER Jr. Emergency therapy of asthma: comparison of the acute effects of parenteral and inhaled sympathomimetics and infused aminophylline. *Am Rev Respir Dis*. 1980;122:365-371.

Schiff GD, Hegde HK, LaCloche L, Hryhorczuk DO. Inpatient theophylline toxicity: preventable factors. *Ann Intern Med*. 1991; 114:748-753.

Stein LM, Cole RP. Early administration of corticosteroids in emergency room treatment of acute asthma. *Ann Intern Med*. 1990;112: 822-827.

Tuxen DV. Detrimental effects of postitive end-expiratory pressure during controlled mechanical ventilation of patients with severe airflow obstruction. *Am Rev Respir Dis*. 1989;140:5-9.

Weiss KB, Wagener DK. Changing patterns of asthma mortality. Identifying target populations at high risk. *JAMA*. 1990;265:1683-1687.

Wrenn K, Slovis CM, Murphy F, Greenberg RS. Aminophylline therapy for acute broncho-spastic disease in the emergency room. *Ann Intern Med*. 1991;115:241-247.

15

16   Special Considerations

The diagnosis and assessment of severity of asthma were discussed in Chapter 5, *Clinical Evaluation and Assessment of Severity*. The differential diagnosis and asthma mimics were reviewed. A number of conditions that may coexist and complicate the management of bronchial asthma will be reviewed in this section (**Table 16.1**). Cardiac disease is well known for producing symptoms that may mimic asthma. When heart disease coexists with asthma, it is essential to optimize left ventricular function and treat congestive heart failure.

Drug-Induced Bronchospasm or Cough

A variety of over-the-counter (OTC) and prescription medications may contribute to acute bronchospasm and/or cough (**Table 16.2**). The respiratory symptoms may be either an isolated response or part of a generalized systemic anaphylaxis. The overall magnitude of drug-induced bronchospasm in the United States remains unknown. Nonsteroidal anti-inflammatory drugs (NSAIDs) are the most common cause of drug-induced asthma. Other agents that have received attention in the literature include:

- Sulfites
- β-Adrenergic blocking agents
- Angiotensin-converting enzyme (ACE) inhibitors
- Tartrazine
- A variety of miscellaneous agents.

16

TABLE 16.1 — Conditions That May Complicate Management of Bronchial Asthma

Comorbid Diseases
- Cardiac disease
- Rhinitis/nasal polyposis/sinusitis
- Drug-induced asthma
- Gastroesophageal reflux disease
- Pulmonary infiltrates
- Allergic bronchopulmonary aspergillosis
- Occupational asthma

Miscellaneous
- Pregnancy
- Perioperative management

The vast majority of the causes of drug-induced asthma are the result of an idiopathic, pharmacologic reaction to a compound. However, other mechanisms include:

- Immunologic, immunoglobulin E (IgE)–requiring mechanism
- Direct, non-IgE related release of mast cell mediators
- Induction of an irritative effect by a variety of cellular mechanisms.

Drug-induced asthma should be suspected in all patients with difficult-to-control or steroid-dependent asthma. Careful history of all prescribed OTC medications should be obtained from all patients with asthma.

■ Aspirin and Nonsteroidal Anti-inflammatory Drugs

Drugs may contribute to perhaps 10% of asthma attacks. About 80% of these episodes of drug-induced asthma are probably secondary to NSAIDs, >50% of which are due to aspirin. There are >200 drugs that contain aspirin. Reported incidence indicates that 5%

to 20% of adults with asthma will experience exacerbations of bronchoconstriction after ingestion of aspirin or other NSAIDs. The prevalence increases with increasing severity of asthma. In a majority of patients with aspirin-induced asthma, the first symptoms appear in the third or fourth decade of life. Over 90% of such patients have associated sinusitis based on radiographic studies. Patients typically have onset of vasomotor rhinitis prior to asthma or aspirin sensitivity. Family history is usually negative in such patients. There is no association between aspirin sensitivity and atopy, since skin tests with common allergens are almost always negative. Also, serum IgE levels are usually normal and specific anti-aspirin IgE antibodies are negative. In these patients, aspirin does not elevate serum IgE levels or the peripheral eosinophil count. The natural history of adult-onset asthma in such patients is generally felt to be quite severe and refractory to therapy. Although there is a statistical correlation between aspirin sensitivity and nasal polyposis, they probably are not causally related. It is likely that aspirin sensitivity, nasal polyps, and sinusitis all increase in prevalence with increasing asthma severity.

Reactions to NSAIDs can be broadly categorized as:
- Mixed rhinoconjunctivitis with bronchospasm
- Pure rhinitis response with urticaria and angioedema.

An adverse reaction to aspirin or NSAIDS may occur at anytime, often following many years of employing these drugs without difficulty. such a reaction is not prevented by pretreatment with antihistamines, theophylline, or cromolyn sodium. Corticosteroids do not prevent the bronchospasm unless given for an extended number of days.

Inhibition of the enzyme cyclooxygenase (COX) is the property that is common to all of the drugs producing this bronchospasm. The severity of bronchospasm

225

TABLE 16.2 — Drugs Implicated in Drug-Induced Bronchospasm or Cough

Drugs That Cross-React in Aspirin-Sensitive Asthma
- Aspirin
- Nonsteroidal anti-inflammatory drugs (NSAIDs):
  - Diclofenac sodium (Voltaren)
  - Ibuprofen (Advil, Motrin)
  - Indomethacin (Indocin)
  - Meclofenamate (Meclomen)
  - Mefenamic acid (Ponstel)
  - Naproxen (Naprosyn, Anaprox)
  - Piroxicam (Feldene)
  - Sulindac (Clinoril)
  - Tolmetin (Tolectin)

Sulfiting Agents

Oral β-Blockers
- Nonselective:
  - Carteolol (Cartrol)*
  - Nadolol
  - Penbutolol (Levatol)*
  - Pindolol (Visken)*
  - Propranolol (Inderal)
  - Sotalol (Betapace)
  - Timolol (Blocadren, Timolide)
- β_1-Selective:
  - Acebutolol (Sectral)*
  - Atenolol (Tenoretic, Tenormin)
  - Betaxolol (Kerlone)
  - Bisoprolol (Zebeta, Ziac)
  - Esmolol (Brevibloc)
  - Metoprolol (Lopressor)
- Combined α-, β-blockade:
  - Carvedilol (Coreg)
  - Labetalol (Normodyne, Trandate)

Angiotensin-Converting Enzyme (ACE) Inhibitors
- First generation
  - Captopril (Capoten)
  - Lisinopril (Prinivil, Zestril)
  - Enalapril (Vasotec)

Continued

Angiotensin-Converting Enzyme (ACE) Inhibitors (cont'd)
- Second generation:
  - Benazepril (Lotensin)
  - Fosinopril (Monopril)
  - Quinapril (Accupril)
  - Ramipril (Altace)
- Third generation:
  - Moexipril (Univasc)
  - Trandolapril (Mavik)

Ophthalmic Agents
- β-Adrenergic blockers:
  - Timolol (Timoptic)
  - Betaxolol (Betoptic)
- Parasympathomimetic drugs:
  - Pilocarpine
  - Carbachol
  - Methacholine
  - Echothiophate
- Other drugs and agents:
  - Anti-inflammatory agents (indomethacin)
  - Sympathomimetic amine (dipivefrin)

* Has intrinsic sympathomimetic activity.

Modified from: Lois M, Honig EG. *J Respir Dis.* 1997;18:569; and, Prakash UB, Rosenow EC III. *Mayo Clin Proc.* 1990;65: 521-529.

appears to be related to a drug's potency as a COX inhibitor. Also, drugs that are not COX inhibitors can be ingested by these patients, even drugs that are structurally similar to aspirin, such as sodium salicylate. Aspirin administration shifts 90% of the arachidonic acid metabolism away from the COX pathway to the 5-lipoxygenase pathway and increases leukotriene production. The sulfidopeptide leukotrienes are well known, potent constrictors of bronchial smooth muscle. Patients with aspirin-sensitive asthma may be ideal candidates for antileukotriene agents. However, why all patients with asthma are not sensitive to aspirin remains unclear.

16

In general, it is recommended that in patients with asthma, aspirin and NSAIDs be used cautiously. If a patient has a history of aspirin-induced asthma, particular care should be taken to counsel the patient of the variety of aspirin-type products to avoid. Patients should be counseled to use alternative products, such as acetaminophen.

If a patient with aspirin-induced asthma has a compelling reason to require therapy with a nonsteroidal agent (ie, therapy for rheumatoid arthritis), oral desensitization may be performed by an experienced physician. In general, reactions to these drugs produce a refractory period lasting 2 to 7 days. These reactions do not occur if patients ingest drugs for an underlying rheumatologic condition on a daily basis. A number of protocols (Pleskow WW et al, 1982) have been published for a graded oral aspirin desensitization.

■ **Tartrazine**

Although early studies have linked the yellow food dye tartrazine (FD&C No. 5) with acute bronchoconstriction and cross-reactivity to aspirin-induced asthma, more recent studies have suggested that tartrazine intolerance is probably rare. Also, tartrazine is not a COX inhibitor, suggesting that if it is associated with bronchospasm, it is not on the basis of cross-reactivity with aspirin sensitivity.

■ **Sulfiting Agents**

Sulfiting agents, including sodium and potassium salts of sulfite, bisulfite, and metabisulfite, are used to preserve foods and beverages and occasionally are used in a variety of oral and parenteral medications. Under certain conditions, these agents liberate sulfur dioxide, which has been well documented to induce acute asthma in susceptible patients. All patients with asthma experience bronchoconstriction on inhaling sulfur dioxide in concentrations greater than one part per million (ppm). However, only a small minority give a classic history of acute worsening of asthma immediately after drinking wine or beer, or unexplained worsening of asthma while eating in restaurants, particularly if the meal included processed potatoes, fresh salads, or fruits. In 1986, the Food and Drug Administration (FDA) banned the use of sulfites on fruits and vegetables served fresh; therefore, there has been a significant reduction in the potential for exposure. Major sources for exposure to sulfites that still may be encountered are:

- Processed potatoes
- Shrimp
- Dried fruits
- Beer
- Wine.

Also, sulfites are contained in:

- Some nebulizer solutions (ie, Bronkosol, Isuprel)
- Injected epinephrine
- Injected lidocaine
- Metoclopramide.

There are no OTC drugs that contain sulfites.

History of adverse reaction to a potential source of sulfite is usually adequate to establish a provisional diagnosis of sulfite sensitivity. A specific diagnosis of sulfite sensitivity requires progressive challenge with solutions containing acidified sulfite. A specific diagnosis should be considered only in patients with a particularly severe reaction. Skin testing or serologic testing is not helpful. Sulfite-sensitive persons should avoid sulfite-treated foods known to trigger the asthmatic response. Inadvertent exposure to sulfites may be treated with subcutaneous epinephrine.

16

■ β-Blocking Agents

A variety of recent practice guidelines have accorded β-blockers an important place in the management of hypertension, as well as post–acute myocardial infarction (MI) care. Data strongly suggest that these agents improve long-term outcome, including survival. These benefits need to be balanced with the well-known bronchospastic adverse effects that occur in patients with asthma and chronic obstructive pulmonary disease (COPD). Other common uses for β-blockers include:

- Migraine headaches
- Idiopathic tremor
- Glaucoma (topical preparation).

In normal individuals, β-blockers do not appear to produce respiratory symptoms, bronchoconstriction, or airway hyperreactivity. In asymptomatic individuals with atopy and family history of asthma, β-blocker use could occasionally bring on bronchospastic symptoms and/or airflow reduction, presumably unmasking underlying asthma. In patients with asthma, a significant percentage (40% to 50%) have wheezing and worsening of indices of airflow. In patients with fixed-airflow obstruction (eg, COPD), this seems to occur in 15% to 20%.

In addition to the underlying disease (asthma or COPD), the relative cardioselectivity of the agent represents the most important risk factor, followed by the presence of intrinsic sympathomimetic activity (ISA). β-Blockers with high affinity for β_1-receptors are referred to as cardioselective. However, selectivity is relative and at high doses any β-blocker can cause blockade of both β_1- and β_2-adrenergic receptors. Data clearly suggest that cardioselective agents (such as atenolol and metoprolol) produce less of a drop in airflow indices compared with nonselective agents.

For patients with airflow obstruction, β-blockers represent a relative contraindication and other agents are generally preferred. However, if benefits of these agents are felt to be substantial (eg, post-acute MI), cardioselective agents are preferred at the lowest dose. Inhaled anticholinergic agents, such as ipratropium, may be particularly useful for β-blockade–induced bronchoconstriction.

■ Angiotensin-Converting Enzyme Inhibitors

A great deal of data exist as to the beneficial effects of ACE inhibitors in patients with hypertension, congestive heart failure, MI, and diabetic nephropathy. Since their introduction, cough has been reported with an incidence of 4% to 30%. The cough:

- Is dry, often starting with a tickle
- Is disabling
- Responds poorly to:
  - Antitussives
  - β-Agonists
  - Inhaled corticosteroids.

Cough may develop anytime after the start of therapy and usually clears within a month after cessation. The cough does not appear to be dose related and it may be seen with any of the available ACE inhibitors.

The mechanism of ACE-induced cough remains speculative. Several reports have suggested an association between ACE-induced cough and underlying bronchial hyperreactivity to methacholine, although this association is not satisfactorily established. Most patients with cough do not have increased bronchial hyperresponsiveness.

Angiotensin-converting enzyme catalyzes the conversion of angiotensin I to angiotensin II. It also inhibits the action of kininase II, which leads to accumulation of:

- Bradykinin
- Substance P
- Prostaglandins.

16

Bradykinin may induce cough and bronchospasm in susceptible persons by stimulating sensory C fibers and phospholipase A_2, which increases production of arachidonic acid metabolites and prostaglandins. Substance P, as a neurotransmitter for C fibers, produces bronchoconstriction. All the available ACE inhibitors, either short- or long-acting, share these properties. Therefore, cough is thought to be a class effect for ACE inhibitors. Data suggest that a person experiencing cough with one ACE inhibitor will most likely experience cough with the others.

Recently, a new class of agents have become available. These agents are known as angiotensin receptor blockers (ARBs). They are selective and do not block the effects of kininase II, thereby not leading to accumulation of bradykinin or substance P. Clinical studies indicate that cough is not a significant side effect with these agents. A recent, randomized study of patients with lisinopril-induced cough compared the effects of losartan (an ARB) with a rechallenge of lisinopril (an ACE inhibitor). The incidence of cough was 18% with losartan and 97% with lisinopril. Currently available ARBs include:

- Candesartan (Atacand)
- Eprosartan (Teveten)
- Irbesartan (Avapro)
- Losartan (Cozaar)
- Olmesartan (Benicar)
- Telmisartan (Micardis)
- Valsartan (Diovan).

In general, cessation of the ACE inhibitor results in resolution of the cough. There have been occasional reports of beneficial effects of a number of agents, including sulindac, cromolyn sodium, and aerosolized lidocaine, in the therapy for ACE-induced cough in the face of ongoing therapy with an ACE inhibitor. Drugs that prevent bradykinin-induced bronchospasm, such as nedocromil sodium, may be useful for treating this type of asthma. ARBs are reasonable alternatives for patients with ACE-inhibitor cough.

Gastroesophageal Reflux Disease

■ **Introduction**

There is substantial literature that suggests a relationship between gastroesophageal reflux disease (GERD) and bronchial asthma. There are several possible associations between these two conditions:

- These are two common diseases that coexist independently in some patients.
- GERD either exacerbates or is causally related to the pathogenesis of asthma in a subset of patients.
- Bronchial asthma and/or antiasthma medications exacerbate or induce GERD.

It is likely that all three of these possibilities occur in subsets of patients with bronchial asthma. The magnitude of the association between GERD and asthma and its clinical significance remains unclear from the literature. GERD, with its primary symptoms of heartburn and acid regurgitation, is common in the general population. A recent, random sample of 2200 Olmstead County residents ages 25 to 74 years found that 20% of the respondents had reflux symptoms at least weekly and nearly 60% had either heartburn or acid regurgitation occurring in the past year. The prevalence of GERD in asthmatics is reported to range from 34% to 89%. Reasons for this wide variability include:

- The use of self-reported questionnaire data
- Comorbid confounding factors, including:
  - Alcohol
  - Cigarette smoking
  - Gender

- The variability of definition and choice of diagnostic techniques to establish GERD.

■ Methodology Issues

A number of methodologic limitations exist in the early, and also more recent, published literature relating GERD and asthma. The major limitation in all the published studies is the lack of attempt to optimize conventional, "standard" therapy for the underlying asthma. Today, this means the use of daily inhaled corticosteroid (ICSs). Inadequate use of ICSs is a major treatment shortcoming for many patients with poorly controlled asthma. Other issues include:

- *The study of a "novel" intervention for GERD-related asthma without instituting conventional asthma therapy* is an important source of variability in the published studies.
- *Lack of objective assessment of acid suppression while asthmatic patients are being treated for GERD*: In the absence of documented control of acid reflux, one cannot conclude that therapy for GERD did not improve the associated asthma.
- *Absence of a control group in some studies*: Based on data from a variety of experimental anti-inflammatory therapies for chronic "steroid-dependent" asthma, it is known that the placebo arm of these asthma studies could improve by 20% to 40% simply by having the subjects participate in a clinical trial, ie, the "Hawthorne effect."
- *Total number of asthmatics subjected to GERD therapy is quite small* (eg, 77 patients in five reports for omeprazole and 125 patients in five reports for H_2-receptor antagonists): Any beneficial effects of antireflux therapy associated with a small improvement in asthma control might not have been detected because of small sample size (β-error).

234

- *Choice of outcome parameters for asthma improvement are inconsistent in the published studies*: The beneficial effect on symptom scores has been much greater than other objective parameters such as peak expiratory flow (PEF) or forced expiratory volume in 1 second (FEV_1).
- *All published trials of therapy for GERD-associated asthma involve asthmatics with symptoms of heartburn or acid regurgitation*: Findings can not be extended to asthmatics with so-called "silent GERD," in which the reflux disease is diagnosed by a positive-pH probe or endoscopic evidence of esophagitis in the absence of GERD symptoms.

Several recently published studies add additional information on the relationship between GERD and asthma, but their results do not completely resolve the questions and issues mentioned above.

A recent, large, prospective cohort study using the UK General Practice Research Database investigated the temporal relationship between asthma and GERD in a general practice setting. A cohort of patients with a first diagnosis of GERD ($n=5653$) and another cohort of patients with a first diagnosis of asthma ($n=9712$) at the initiation of the study were compared with age-matched and gender-matched control cohorts without either diagnosis. All cohorts were followed for a mean of 3 years. The incidence rates of GERD and asthma among the control cohorts were 4.4 and 3.8 per 1000 person-years, respectively. During the follow-up period, the relative risk (RR) of an incident asthma diagnosis in patients with a first diagnosis of GERD was 1.2 (95% confidence interval [CI], 0.9 to 1.6), while the RR of an incident GERD diagnosis among patients with a first diagnosis of asthma was 1.5 (95% CI, 1.2 to 1.8) after adjustment for age, gender, smoking, prior

16

comorbidity, and number of health care contacts. The increase in risk was mainly seen during the first year of follow-up. The prior use of prescription medications for asthma and GERD had no significant effects on the subsequent risk of GERD or asthma, respectively. The investigators concluded that patients with asthma are at a significantly increased risk for developing GERD, mainly during the first years following diagnosis, whereas patients with GERD have a nonsignificant risk of developing asthma.

Another recent study sought to determine the prevalence of GERD, as indicated by both symptoms and objective evidence (eg, 24-hour dual-probe pH monitoring), in 68 patients with difficult-to-control asthma attending a "difficult asthma" clinic. The prevalence of GERD/GERD-associated asthma symptoms was 75% (95% CI, 63% to 84.7%). The prevalence of GERD as evidenced by an abnormal pH profile at the distal esophageal probe was 55%, while the pH profile was abnormal at the proximal probe in 34.6% of patients. Asymptomatic GERD was present in 9.6% of patients; 16% of cough episodes correlated with acid reflux. The presence of GERD was similar in difficult-to-control asthmatic patients who had responded to interventions and those in whom their asthma remained difficult to control.

■ Medical Treatment

The primary goal of managing GERD with or without associated extraesophageal disease is complete symptom resolution. Additional therapeutic end points include:

- Healing of esophagitis when present
- Prevention of complications, such as peptic stricture or Barrett's esophagus
- Maintenance of symptom control in patients with chronic disease.

The overall management strategies can be classified as:

- Lifestyle changes
- Pharmacologic manipulations of gastric acid and motility
- Surgery.

See **Table 16.3** for a summary of antireflux medications.

■ Proposed Approach to GERD-Associated Asthma

Our approach to GERD in asthmatics is summarized in **Figure 16.1**. We favor an aggressive empiric therapy for both GERD and asthma, with judicious use of diagnostic studies. For patients with suboptimal control of asthma, based on frequent symptoms, daily use of bronchodilators, need for prednisone bursts and

---

TABLE 16.3 — Antireflux Medications for the Treatment of GERD
Antacids
Alginic Acid (Gaviscon)
H₂-Receptor Antagonists • Cimetidine (Tagamet) • Famotidine (Pepcid) • Nizatidine (Axid) • Ranitidine (Zantac)
Prokinetic Agents • Metoclopramide (Reglan) • Bethanechol (Urecholine) • Domperidone maleate (Motilium)
H⁺/K⁺-ATPase (proton pump) Inhibitors • Omeprazole (Prilosec) • Lansoprazole (Prevacid) • Pantoprazole (Protonix) • Esomeprazole (Nexium) • Rabeprazole (Aciphex)

16

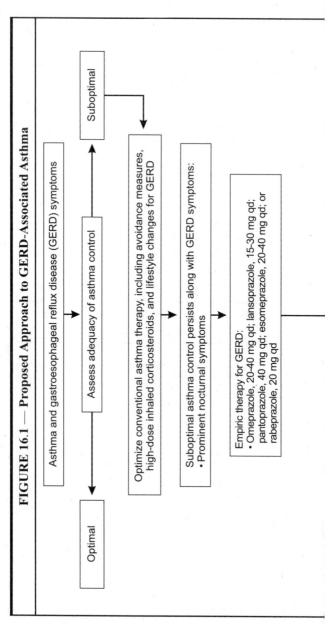

FIGURE 16.1 — Proposed Approach to GERD-Associated Asthma

Asthma and gastroesophageal reflux disease (GERD) symptoms

Assess adequacy of asthma control

Optimal

Suboptimal

Optimize conventional asthma therapy, including avoidance measures, high-dose inhaled corticosteroids, and lifestyle changes for GERD

Suboptimal asthma control persists along with GERD symptoms:
• Prominent nocturnal symptoms

Empiric therapy for GERD:
• Omeprazole, 20-40 mg qd; lansoprazole, 15-30 mg qd; pantoprazole, 40 mg qd; esomeprazole, 20-40 mg qd; or rabeprazole, 20 mg qd

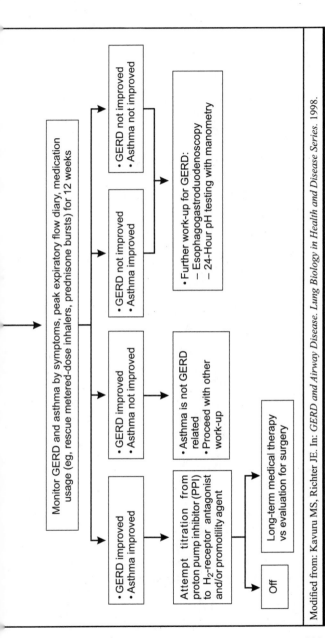

Monitor GERD and asthma by symptoms, peak expiratory flow diary, medication usage (eg, rescue metered-dose inhalers, prednisone bursts) for 12 weeks

- GERD improved
- Asthma improved

Attempt titration from proton pump inhibitor (PPI) to H₂-receptor antagonist and/or promotility agent

- Long-term medical therapy vs evaluation for surgery
- Off

- GERD improved
- Asthma not improved

- Asthma is not GERD related
- Proceed with other work-up

- GERD not improved
- Asthma improved

- GERD not improved
- Asthma not improved

- Further work-up for GERD:
  – Esophagogastroduodenoscopy
  – 24-Hour pH testing with manometry

Modified from: Kavuru MS, Richter JE. In: *GERD and Airway Disease. Lung Biology in Health and Disease Series.* 1998.

16

239

emergency visits, we carefully optimize conventional asthma therapy. Based on consensus guidelines, this would include:

- Patient education
- Trigger-avoidance measures
- Appropriate use of PEF monitoring
- Daily inhaled corticosteroids (ICSs) in appropriate doses.

For patients who continue to have poor asthma control, a careful investigation is pursued to exclude asthma mimics and search for comorbid disease or exacerbating factors, including:

- Environmental allergies
- Chronic nasal and sinus disease:
  – Rhinitis
  – Polyposis
  – Sinusitis
- Pulmonary infiltrates
- GERD.

For patients who have symptomatic GERD, and perhaps prominent nocturnal symptoms, we recommend specific lifestyle changes and empiric therapy with proton pump inhibitors (PPIs), 12-week trial at a dosage of 20-40 mg qd for omeprazole, 15-30 mg qd with lansoprazole, 40 mg qd with pantoprazole, 20-40 mg qd with esomeprazole, or 20 mg qd with rabeprazole. We subsequently monitor both GERD and asthma by:

- Symptoms
- PEF diary
- Rescue medication use.

The outcome of this intervention could fall into one of four groups (**Figure 16.1**). Both GERD and asthma may be improved, which would suggest that GERD is an important trigger. In this subset, the next challenge is long-term management, including gradual titration from proton pump inhibition to H_2-receptor antagonist and/or promotility drug, long-term PPI therapy, or evaluation for surgery. GERD may be improved, but asthma may remain unchanged, suggesting that GERD is not an important trigger. If GERD is not improved with an empiric trial of PPI, further work-up should include specific diagnostic studies, such as pH testing with manometry and endoscopy, to ensure that acid reflux has been adequately controlled.

There have been several recent, large, randomized, placebo-controlled studies of the effects of treatment of GERD with PPIs in patients with asthma. Again, there are some issues with methodology and the results, although promising, are less than conclusive.

The effects of 24 weeks' treatment with lansoprazole 30 mg bid were assessed in a multicenter, double-blind, randomized, placebo-controlled trial in 207 patients with moderate-to-severe asthma receiving usual asthma care, including ICSs. Daily asthma symptoms, albuterol use, PEF, FEV_1, forced vital capacity (FVC), and investigator-assessed symptoms at 24 weeks, did not improve significantly with lansoprazole treatment compared with placebo. The emotional function of domain of the Asthma Quality of Life with Standardized Activities Questionnaire (AQLQS) improved significantly ($P = 0.025$) at 24 weeks with lansoprazole. Compared with placebo, fewer patients receiving lansoprazole (8.1% vs 20.4%, $P = 0.017$) experienced exacerbations and oral corticosteroid-treated exacerbations of asthma (4% vs 13.9%, $P = 0.016$).

A 16-week, randomized, double-blind, placebo-controlled trial in 770 patients with or without GERD, but with persistent moderate-to-severe asthma receiving anti-inflammatory asthma medications compared the effects of esomeprazole 40 mg bid and placebo on lung function and nocturnal respiratory symptoms (NOC). According to the presence or absence of NOC

16

and GERD, patients were divided into three strata: GERD–/NOC+, GERD+/NOC–, and GERD+ /NOC+. In the overall study population, the improvement in morning PEF in esomeprazole-treated patients (6.3 L/min) was not significantly different ($P = 0.061$) from that in placebo-treated patients. However, in GERD+/NOC+ patients ($n=350$), esomeprazole provided an 8.7 L/min improvement ($P = 0.3$) in morning PEF and a 10.2 L/min improvement ($P = 0.012$) in evening PEF compared with placebo. In patients receiving long-acting β_2-agonists ($n=307$), even greater improvements in morning PEF (12.2 L/min, $P = 0.017$) and evening PEF (11.1 L/min, $P = 0.024$) were observed in esomeprazole-treated patients; these improvements were more pronounced in GERD+/NOC+ patients.

■ Pulmonary Infiltrates and Bronchial Asthma

Occasionally, the clinical course of a patient with bronchial asthma may be complicated by pulmonary parenchymal infiltrates apparent on the chest radiograph. The differential diagnosis for an infiltrate is extensive. However, specific entities to consider in an asthmatic include:

- Typical and atypical infections
- Allergic bronchopulmonary aspergillosis (ABPA)
- Chronic eosinophilic pneumonia and other pulmonary infiltrate with eosinophilia (PIE) syndromes
- Allergic granulomatosis with angiitis (Churg-Strauss syndrome).

Discussion here will be limited to ABPA.

Allergic bronchopulmonary aspergillosis appears to complicate 1% to 2% of all cases of chronic asthma. ABPA is an entity distinct from a variety of other Aspergillus-related respiratory diseases such as:

- Invasive aspergillosis

- Aspergilloma
- Hypersensitivity pneumonitis
- Semi-invasive aspergillosis with chronic necrotizing pneumonia.

ABPA represents a colonization of the lungs associated with a particular host-immunologic response. It is important to note that ABPA is not an infection; therefore, it is not treatable with antifungal therapy. A variety of diagnostic features are often present in this entity and are listed in **Table 16.4**. Not all of these features need to be present at one time. Patients with ABPA characteristically have fleeting pulmonary infiltrates and central bronchiectasis in the setting of difficult-to-control bronchial asthma. In general, oral corticosteroids are the treatment of choice for ABPA. Greenberger and Patterson recommend prednisone at 0.5 mg/kg/day given as a single morning dose for 2 weeks, then converted to an alternate-day dosing schedule for a total of 3 months of therapy. The drug is subsequently tapered and eventually discontinued. Some have also recommended titrating therapy to total serum IgE values. As mentioned earlier, antifungal agents administered either systemically or by the nebulized route have not been shown to be effective for ABPA.

TABLE 16.4 — Diagnostic Features of Allergic Bronchopulmonary Aspergillosis

- Asthma
- Pulmonary infiltrate(s)
- Central bronchiectasis
- Immediate cutaneous reactivity to the *Aspergillus* species (prick or intradermal)
- Elevated total serum IgE level
- Peripheral blood eosinophilia
- Precipitating antibodies to *A fumigatus*
- Elevated serum IgE and/or IgG for *A fumigatus*

16

Occupational asthma can be loosely defined as episodic respiratory symptoms with reversible airflow obstruction and increased airway reactivity that is caused by exposure to substances in the workplace. Occupational asthma should be differentiated from preexisting bronchial asthma that is exacerbated in a nonspecific manner in the workplace. Currently, occupational asthma is the most common occupational lung disease. An estimated 2% of all asthma cases may be of occupational origin. Over 200 asthma-causing agents have been identified in the workplace; **Table 16.5** is a partial list.

Occupational asthma is often classified as either allergic or nonallergic. The allergic occupational asthma is characterized by the presence of latency and specific airway hyperresponsiveness. This type of asthma is usually characterized by a preceding latent period, during which exposure occurs without symptoms. Allergic sensitization occurs in the workplace, and when challenged with the specific agent in the laboratory, an immunologically mediated late-phase response occurs. Allergic occupational asthma typically involves high molecular-weight agents (>1000 daltons) such as:

- Animal proteins
- Enzymes
- Vegetable matter.

Also, atopy may be an important risk factor for this type of asthma. These features of latency and specific immunologic hyperresponsiveness are absent in non-allergic occupational asthma, which is usually caused by low molecular-weight agents. Both allergic and non-allergic occupational asthma are characterized by the presence of nonspecific airway hyperresponsiveness (as assessed by methacholine or histamine provocation) and airway inflammation.

Occupational asthma is most often determined by obtaining a careful history. Typical symptoms are those of bronchial asthma and include:

- Cough
- Wheeze
- Chest tightness
- Dyspnea.

These symptoms tend to improve or resolve during extended periods away from the workplace, such as on weekends and on vacation, and are the most important features of the history. Symptoms may initially be present at the workplace and worsen during the latter portion of the workweek. With chronic exposure, symptoms may be more prominent in the evening hours or 12 hours after the work shift. Objective assessment of airflow obstruction at the workplace is essential.

The use of a peak-flow meter every 1 to 2 hours during both working and nonworking days for 2 to 4 weeks is essential. Variability in PEF of >20% during work or in the evening hours would strongly suggest a diagnosis of occupational asthma. Occasionally, inhalation challenge with agents suspected of causing occupational asthma is conducted if the diagnosis remains in question or if there are medicolegal issues for compensation or disability. This should only be conducted by experienced specialists familiar with the technique.

Pregnancy and Asthma 16

During pregnancy, asthma is the most common pulmonary disease requiring physician intervention. It is estimated that approximately 1% of pregnancies are complicated by asthma. In one of every 500 of these pregnancies, asthma is severe and life-threatening.

TABLE 16.5 — Asthma-Causing Agents in Selected Occupations

Occupation/Occupational Field	Agent
Animal Proteins	
Laboratory animal workers, veterinarians	Dander and urine proteins
Food processing	Shellfish, egg proteins, pancreatic enzymes, amylase
Dairy farmers	Storage mites
Poultry farmers	Poultry mites, droppings, and feathers
Research workers	Locusts
Fish-food manufacturing	Midges
Detergent manufacturing	*Bacillus subtilis* enzymes
Silk workers	Silk-worm moths and larvas
Plant Proteins	
Bakers	Flour
Food processing	Coffee bean dust, meat tenderizer (papain), tea
Farmers	Soy bean dust
Shipping workers	Grain dust (molds, insects, grain)
Laxative manufacturing	Ispaghula

Sawmill workers, carpenters	Wood dust (western red cedar, oak, mahogany, zebrawood, red wood, Lebanon cedar, African maple, eastern white cedar)
Granary workers	Storage mites, *Aspergillus*, indoor ragweed, and grass pollen
Electric soldering	Colophony (pine resin)
Cotton textile workers	Cotton dust
Nurses	Psyllium
Inorganic Chemicals	
Refining	Platinum salts
Plating	Nickel salts
Diamond polishing	Cobalt salts
Stainless steel welding	Chromium salts
Manufacturing	Aluminum fluoride
Beauty shop	Persulfate
Refinery workers	Vanadium
Welding	Stainless steel fumes

Continued

16

247

Occupation/Occupational Field	Agent
	Organic Chemicals
Manufacturing	Antibiotics, piperazine, methyldopa, salbutamol, cimetidine
Hospital workers	Disinfectants (sulfathiazole, chloramine, formaldehyde, psyllium, glutaraldehyde)
Anesthesiology	Enflurane
Poultry workers	Amprolium
Fur dyeing	Paraphenylene diamine
Rubber processing	Formaldehyde, ethylene diamine, phthalic anhydride
Plastics industry	Toluene diisocyanate, hexamethyl diisocyanate, dephenyl-methyl isocyanate, phthalic anhydride, triethylene tetramines, trimellitic anhydride, hexamethyl tetramine
Automobile painting	Dimethyl ethanolamine, toluene diisocyanate
Foundry worker	Furfuryl, alcohol resin

Modified from: *Clinical Practice Guidelines. Expert Panel Report 2: Guidelines for the Diagnosis and Management of Asthma.* Bethesda, Md: US Dept of Health and Human Services; 1997. NIH publication 97-4051.

Prevention of asthma attacks, and aggressive and optimal management of exacerbations are imperative for the health of both the mother and the fetus. Broadly speaking, there are three issues:

- The impact of pregnancy on preexisting asthma as to its relative control.
- The impact of asthma on the outcome of the pregnancy for both the mother and the fetus.
- The relative safety concerning the health of the fetus of a variety of medications that may be used for asthma and allergic rhinitis.

Review of a large number of studies suggests that the course of asthma during pregnancy is quite variable. It appears that patients with mild asthma may improve during pregnancy, whereas patients with severe asthma tend to have exacerbations during pregnancy. Also, exacerbations tend to occur more often during the end of the second trimester. Severe exacerbations during labor are apparently rare. Within the first 3 months postpartum, the asthma severity tends to revert to the prepregnant level. A number of studies suggest that an individual is likely to have a similar clinical course of asthma control during subsequent pregnancies.

An early study showed a 2-fold increase in maternal complications (toxemia, postpartum hemorrhage, and hyperemesis gravidarum) in asthmatic women during pregnancy. However, most modern studies suggest that asthmatic pregnancies are not associated with an increased risk of prematurity or perinatal mortality if maternal asthma is under proper control during the gestational period. Infants of asthmatic mothers do appear to have a higher incidence of low birth weight. For a variety of reasons, poor asthma control leads to suboptimal fetal outcome. Many studies also suggest that pregnant asthmatics are also more likely to receive epidural analgesia and have a cesarean section than

16

are nonasthmatic subjects. However, these are largely retrospective and uncontrolled studies.

The potential therapeutic benefit of any drug used in pregnancy must be weighed against any possible harmful maternal or fetal side effects. Drugs typically used for the management of asthma are generally safe during pregnancy. In general, it is felt that optimal control of asthma with the fewest exacerbations has greater benefit than the potential adverse effects of asthma medications on the fetus. The approach to drug therapy in pregnancy is much the same as chronic care for asthma in any patient. In general, inhaled medications are preferred to oral or parenteral agents. Early institution of systemic corticosteroid therapy is preferred for acute exacerbations.

The FDA has published guidelines for prescribing asthma medications to pregnant women. Drugs are classified into four groups (groups A through D) based on the available data on the relative risk. Most asthma medications are classified as group B or C. The drugs classified as group D should not be prescribed to pregnant asthmatics, including:

- Tetracycline
- Iodide-containing expectorants.

These medications and FDA risk-factor ratings are summarized in **Table 16.6** and **Table 16.7**.

Perioperative Management of Asthma

Data suggest that 3.5% of patients presenting for anesthesia suffer from bronchial asthma. Asthmatic patients are more likely to have both operative and postoperative pulmonary complications. Preoperative evaluation of an asthmatic includes the following issues:

- Assess the severity and overall control of asthma.

TABLE 16.6 — Risk of Allergy and Asthma Medications in First Trimester of Pregnancy			
Drug	No. of Patients Exposed	Standardized Risk*	Significance
Corticosteroids	145	0.67	—
Tripelennamine	100	0.81	—
Isoproterenol	31	0.94	—
Atropine	401	1.04	—
Ephedrine	373	1.07	—
Chlorpheniraminea	1070	1.20	—
Diphenhydramine	595	1.25	—
Phenylephrine	1249	1.31	< 0.05
Theophylline	117	1.38	—
Phenylpropanolamine	726	1.40	< 0.01
Hydroxyzine	50	1.44	—
Epinephrine	189	1.71	< 0.05
Brompheniramine	65	2.34	< 0.05

* Normalized risk is 1.00.

Clinical Practice Guidelines. Expert Panel Report 2: Guidelines for the Diagnosis and Management of Asthma. Bethesda, Md: US Dept of Health and Human Services; 1997. NIH publication 97-4051.

16

TABLE 16.7 – Risk to Fetus of Allergy and Asthma Medications During Pregnancy

	Risk Factor Category
Bronchodilator	
Terbutaline	B
Albuterol	C
Metaproterenol	C
Salmeterol	C
Theophylline	C
Anti-inflammatory	
Cromolyn sodium	B
Montelukast	B
Nedocromil sodium	B
Zafirlukast	B
Beclomethasone dipropionate	C
Budesonide	C
Flunisolide	C
Fluticasone	C
Mometasone	C
Triamcinolone	C
Zileuton	C
Prednisone	(Not rated)
Antihistamine	
Chlorpheniramine	B
Triprolidine	B
Astemizole	C
Brompheniramine	C
Terfenadine	C

Key to Risk-Factor Ratings
(According to Manufacturer's FDA-Approved Product Labeling)

A **Controlled studies show no risk**. Adequate, well-controlled studies in pregnant women have failed to demonstrate risk to the fetus.

B **No evidence of risk in humans**. Either animal findings show risk, but human findings do not; or, if no adequate human studies have been done, animal findings are negative.

C **Risk cannot be ruled out**. Human studies are lacking, and animal studies are either positive for fetal risk or lacking as well. However, potential benefits may justify the potential risk.

D **Positive evidence of risk**. Investigational or postmarketing data show risk to the fetus. Nevertheless, potential benefits may outweigh the potential risk.

X **Contraindicated in pregnancy**. Studies in animals or humans, or investigational or postmarketing reports, have shown fetal risk that clearly outweighs any possible benefit to the patient.

Modified from: *Clinical Practice Guidelines. Expert Panel Report 2: Guidelines for the Diagnosis and Management of Asthma.* Bethesda, Md: US Dept of Health and Human Services; 1997. NIH publication 97-4051.

- Assess the risk of anesthesia for the particular type of surgery.
- Institute perioperative interventions to minimize risk.

Overall, asthmatics are at increased risk for perioperative complications for several reasons:

- Acute airflow obstruction causes ventilation-perfusion mismatching and this may contribute to hypoxemia and hypercapnia, which are reversible.
- Endotracheal intubation and manipulation may trigger or exacerbate bronchospasm.
- Certain medications that may be used in the perioperative period may contribute to bronchospasm.
- Severe airflow obstruction, in conjunction with postoperative pain and the associated sedation, can impair cough with subsequent risk for:
  - Atelectasis
  - Mucous plugging
  - Nosocomial pneumonia.

The clinical evaluation of asthma severity has been reviewed previously. In general, elective surgery should be postponed for patients with active asthma with daily symptoms who are submaximally treated. In fact, active bronchospasm and hypercapnia are absolute contraindications for elective surgery since they are potentially reversible. All patients should receive both preoperative and postoperative inhaled ß-agonists. In addition, almost all patients should also receive preoperative systemic corticosteroids to minimize the risk of active asthma during the induction process. For an otherwise stable asthmatic on chronic maintenance inhaled therapy, preoperative prednisone therapy at 40 mg/day for 2 days before the surgery and 40 mg on the morning of the surgery by mouth is

16

adequate. For patients with particularly severe asthma, hospitalization for a day or more prior to surgery may be recommended for optimization of lung function by aggressive inhaled β-agonists and intravenous corticosteroids. Finally, patients with asthma who have taken systemic corticosteroids in the past 6 months and whose asthma is currently well controlled, may be at risk for depressed adrenal-pituitary response to stress, and perioperative corticosteroid prophylaxis is generally the practice (ie, hydrocortisone 100 mg pre-, intra-, and postoperative).

For patients with asthma, modification of the anesthetic approach by avoiding endotracheal intubation is preferable, if possible by the spinal, epidural, or local anesthesia route. Also, a number of agents are generally not recommended in patients with asthma because of fear of exacerbating bronchospasm. These agents include:

- Morphine
- Meperidine
- D-Tubocurarine
- Ester-type local anesthetics.

In general, induction agents that are acceptable include:

- Barbiturates
- Maintenance inhalational anesthetics, such as halothane and isoflurane
- Muscle relaxants, such as succinylcholine.

Many of the agents have effects on the myocardium, and this should be kept in mind, especially with concomitant use of inhaled β-agonists and aminophylline.

SUGGESTED READING

Drug-Induced Bronchospasm or Cough

ACC/AHA guidelines for the management of patients with acute myocardial infarction. A report of the American College of Cardiology/American Heart Association Task Force on Practice Guidelines (Committee on Management of Acute Myocardial Infarction). *J Am Coll Cardiol.* 1996;28:1328-1428.

Bucknall CE, Neilly JB, Carter R, Stevenson RD, Semple PF. Bronchial hyperreactivity in patients who cough after receiving angiotensin converting enzyme inhibitors. *Br Med J.* 1988;296:86-88.

Chan P, Tomlinson B, Huang TY, Ko JT, Lin TS, Lee YS. Double-blind comparison of losartan, lisinopril, and metolazone in elderly hypertensive patients with previous angiotensin-converting enzyme inhibitor-induced cough. *J Clin Pharmacol.* 1997;37:253-257.

Hannaway PJ, Hopper GD. Severe anaphylaxis and drug-induced beta-blockade. *N Engl J Med.* 1983;308:1536.

Lois M, Honig EG. Beta-blockade post-MI: safe for patients with asthma or COPD. *J Respir Dis.* 1997;18:568-591.

Martinez EJ, Seleznick MJ. Respiratory tract side effects of angiotensin converting enzyme inhibitors: current knowledge. *South Med J.* 1991;84:1343-1346.

Meeker DP, Wiedemann HP. Drug-induced bronchospasm. *Clin Chest Med.* 1990;11:163-175.

Moser M. Angiotensin-converting enzyme inhibitors, angiotensin II receptor antagonists and calcium channel blocking agents: a review of potential benefits and possible adverse reactions. *J Am Coll Cardiol.* 1997;29:1414-1421.

Pleskow WW, Stevenson DD, Mathison DA, Simon RA, Schatz M, Zeiger RS. Aspirin desensitization in aspirin-sensitive asthmatic patients: clinical manifestations and characterization of the refractory period. *J Allergy Clin Immunol.* 1982;69:11-19.

Pleskow WW, Stevenson DD, Mathison DA, Simon RA, Schatz M, Zeiger RS. Aspirin-sensitive rhinosinusitis/asthma: spectrum of adverse reactions to aspirin. *J Allergy Clin Immunol.* 1983;71:574-579.

Prakash UB, Rosenow EC 3rd. Pulmonary complications from ophthalmic preparations. *Mayo Clin Proc.* 1990;65:521-529.

16

Slepian IK, Mathews KP, McLean JA. Aspirin-sensitive asthma. *Chest*. 1985;87:386-391.

Stoller JK, Elghazawi A, Mehta AC, Vidt DG. Captopril-induced cough. *Chest*. 1988;93:659-661.

Gastroesophageal Reflux Disease

Bocskei C, Viczian M, Bocskei R, Horvath I. The influence of gastroesophageal reflux disease and its treatment on asthmatic cough. *Lung*. 2005;183:53-62.

Calabrese C, Fabbri A, Areni A, Scialpi C, Zahlane D, Di Febo G. Asthma and gastroesophageal reflux disease: effect of long-term pantoprazole therapy. *World J Gastroenterol*. 2005;11:7657-7660.

Harding SM, Richter JE. The role of gastroesophageal reflux in chronic cough and asthma. *Chest*. 1997;111:1389-1402.

Kahrilas PJ, Quigley EM. Clinical esophageal pH recording: a technical review for practice guideline development. *Gastroenterology*. 1996;110:1982-1996.

Kavuru MS, Richter JE. Medical treatment of gastroesophageal reflux disease and airway disease. In: Stein MR, ed. *GERD and Airway Disease. Lung Biology in Health and Disease Series*. NY: Marcell Dekker, Inc; 1998.

Kiljander TO, Harding SM, Field SK, et al. Effects of esomeprazole 40 mg twice daily on asthma: a randomized placebo-controlled trial. *Am J Respir Crit Care Med*. 2006;173:1091-1097.

Legget JJ, Johnston BT, Mills M, Gamble J, Heaney LG. Prevalence of gastroesophageal reflux in difficult asthma: relationship to asthma outcome. *Chest*. 2005;127:1227-1231.

Littner MR, Leung FW, Ballard ED 2nd, Huang B, Samra NK; Lansoprazole Asthma Study Group. Effects of 24 weeks of lansoprazole therapy on asthma symptoms, exacerbations, quality of life, and pulmonary function in adult asthmatic patients with acid reflux symptoms. *Chest*. 2005;128:1128-1135.

Ruigomez A, Rodriguez LA, Wallander MA, Johansson S, Thomas M, Price D. Gastroesophageal reflux disease and asthma: a longitudinal study in UK general practice. *Chest*. 2005;128:85-93.

Simpson WG. Gastroesophageal reflux disease and asthma. Diagnosis and management. *Arch Intern Med*. 1995;155:798-803.

Stordal K, Johannesdottir GB, Bentsen BS, et al. Acid suppression does not change respiratory symptoms in children with asthma and gastro-oesophageal reflux disease. *Arch Dis Child*. 2005;90:956-960.

Yuksel H, Yilmaz O, Kirmaz C, Aydogdu S, Kasirga E. Frequency of gastroesophageal reflux disease in nonatopic children with asthma-like airway disease. *Respir Med*. 2006;100:393-398.

Vigneri S, Termini R, Leandro G, et al. A comparison of five maintenance therapies for reflux esophagitis. *N Engl J Med*. 1995;333: 1106-1110.

Occupational Asthma
Alberts WM, Brooks SM. Advances in occupational asthma. *Clin Chest Med*. 1992;13:281-302.

Chan-Yeung M. Evaluation of impairment/disability in patients with occupational asthma. *Am Rev Respir Dis*. 1987;135:950-951.

Evaluation of impairment/disability secondary to respiratory disorders. American Thoracic Society. *Am Rev Respir Dis*. 1986;133: 1205-1209.

Fine JM, Balmes JR. Airway inflammation and occupational asthma. *Clin Chest Med*. 1988;9:577-590.

Malo JL, Ghezzo H, L'Archevêque J, Lagier F, Perrin B, Cartier A. Is the clinical history a satisfactory means of diagnosing occupational asthma? *Am Rev Respir Dis*. 1991;143:528-532.

Mapp CE, Boschetto P, Dal Vecchio L, Maestrelli P, Fabbri LM. Occupational asthma due to isocyanates. *Eur Respir J*. 1988;1:273-279.

Smith DD. Medical-legal definition of occupational asthma. *Chest*. 1990;98:1007-1011.

Tarlo SM, Broder I. Irritant-induced occupational asthma. *Chest*. 1989;96:297-300.

16

Perioperative Management of Asthma
Geiger KK, Hedley-Whyte J. Preoperative and postoperative considerations. In: Weiss EB, Stein M, eds. *Bronchial Asthma: Mechanisms and Therapeutics*. 3rd ed. Boston, Mass: Little Brown & Co; 1993:1099-1113.

Gold MI, Ravin MB. Anesthesia for the asthmatic patient. In: Ravin MB, ed. *Problems in Anesthesia: A Case Study Approach*. Boston, Mass: Little Brown & Co; 1981:29-36.

Pulmonary Infiltrates and Bronchial Asthma

Greenberger PA, Patterson R. Diagnosis and management of allergic bronchopulmonary aspergillosis. *Ann Allergy*. 1986;56:444-448.

Paganin F, Trussard V, Seneterre E, et al. Chest radiography and high resolution computed tomography of the lungs in asthma. *Am Rev Respir Dis*. 1992;146:1084-1087.

Rosenberg M, Patterson R, Mintzer R, Cooper BJ, Roberts M, Harris KE. Clinical and immunologic criteria for the diagnosis of allergic bronchopulmonary aspergillosis. *Ann Intern Med*. 1977;86:405-414.

Pregnancy and Asthma

Apter AJ, Greenberger PA, Patterson R. Outcomes of pregnancy in adolescents with severe asthma. *Arch Intern Med*. 1989;149:2571-2575.

Fitzsimons R, Greenberger PA, Patterson R. Outcome of pregnancy in women requiring corticosteroids for severe asthma. *J Allergy Clin Immunol*. 1986;78:349-353.

Greenberger PA, Patterson R. Current concepts. Management of asthma during pregnancy. *N Engl J Med*. 1985;312:897-902.

National Asthma Education Program Report of the Working Group on Asthma and Pregnancy. *Management of Asthma During Pregnancy*. Bethesda, Md; US Dept of Health and Human Services, Public Health Service, National Institutes of Health; 1993. NIH publication 93-3779.

Schatz M. Asthma and pregnancy. *Immunol Allergy Clin North Am*. 1996;16:893-916.

Schatz M, Zeiger RS. Treatment of asthma and allergic rhinitis during pregnancy. *Ann Allergy*. 1990;65:427-429.

Stenius-Aarniala B, Piirila P, Teramo K. Asthma and pregnancy: a prospective study of 198 pregnancies. *Thorax*. 1988;43:12-18.

Venkataraman MT, Shanies HM. Pregnancy and asthma. *J Asthma*. 1997;34:265-271.

17 Appendix

Organizations and Resources for Asthma:
Educational Materials and Information

Allergy & Asthma Network Mothers
of Asthmatics, Inc. (AANMA)
2751 Prosperity Ave, Suite 150
Fairfax, VA 22031
Phone: 800/878-4403
Fax: 703/573-7794
Web site: www.aanma.org/headquarters

A nonprofit organization founded in 1985 to help families in their quest to overcome and maintain control of asthma, allergies and related conditions. AAN/MA produces *The MA Report*, a monthly newsletter for family education. A wide variety of books and videos are available from the learning resource center.

American Academy of Allergy,
Asthma & Immunology (AAAAI)
555 East Wells Street, Suite 1100
Milwaukee, WI 53202-3823
Phone: 800/822-2762 or 414/272-6071
Web site: www.aaaai.org

Publishes *Asthma and Allergy ADVOCATE*; the toll-free number can be used for physician referral and information. The AAAAI offers brochures, booklets, newsletters and videos; additional booklets are available for schools and nebulizer school nurses.

American Academy of Pediatrics (AAP)
141 Northwest Point Blvd.
Elk Grove Village, IL 60007-1098
Phone: 847/434-4000
Fax: 847/434-8000
Web site: www.aap.org

Brochures on asthma/allergy are available, as well as information regarding children with allergies and asthma, clinical guidelines, asthma triggers, using peak flow meters for monitoring asthma, and understanding asthma. Resources are available for health care professionals.

American Association for Respiratory Care (AARC)
9425 N MacArthur Blvd, Suite 100
Irving, TX 75063-4706
Phone: 972/243-2272
FAX: 972/484-2720 or 972/484-6010
E-mail: info@aarc.org
Web site: www.aarc.org
    National organization of respiratory therapists. Offers a free peak-
    flow based program for schools, *Peak Performance USA*.

American College of Allergy, Asthma
& Immunology (ACAAI)
85 West Algonquin Road, Suite 550
Arlington Heights, IL 60005
Phone: 847/427-1200
Fax: 847/427-1294
Web site: www.acaai.org
    Booklets and other materials on allergies and asthma; most
    information in booklets and other materials appear on the web
    site. The toll-free number may be used for ordering booklets and
    materials on asthma and a list of allergists by state. ACAI provides
    educational materials and forms for use in schools. They also
    sponsor regional asthma education conferences for the public. The
    Web site is maintained by allergists, the medical specialists who
    treat allergies and asthma, and their professional association, the
    American College of Allergy, Asthma & Immunology.

American College of Chest Physicians (ACCP)
3300 Dundee Road
Northbrook, IL 60062
Phone: 847/498-1400 or 800/343-2227
Fax: 847/498-5450
Web site: www.chestnet.org
    Brochures on asthma are available for patients and health care
    professionals. Patient instructions for inhaled devices are included
    on this web site, as well as practice resources for clinicians.

American Lung Association (ALA)
61 Broadway, 6th Floor
New York, NY 10006
Phone: 212/315-8700 or 800/586-4872
Web site: www.lungusa.org
    Local chapters may be contacted for information and booklets
    on lung health. The *Breathe Easy/Asthma Digest* brings the latest
    asthma research and news items right to your electronic mailbox
    each month. There is no charge for this service. Sign up on ALA
    Web site. *The Weekly Breather* is the ALA's weekly electronic

summary of issues in the news related to lung disease and health. The Weekly Breather brings you abstracts of items from major newspapers on topics including asthma. There is no charge for this service. Sign up on the ALA Web site.

American Thoracic Society (ATS)
61 Broadway
New York, NY 10006-2755
Phone: 212/315-8600
Web site: www.thoracic.org

The ATS focuses on respiratory and critical care medicine. The web site contains information about education, meetings, courses, and membership for professionals.

Association of Asthma Educators (AAE)
1215 Anthony Avenue
Columbia, SC 29201-1701
Phone: 888/988-7747
Web site: www.asthmaeducators.org

The primary purpose of the AAE is to promote asthma education as an integral comprehensive asthma program, to raise the competence of health care professionals who educate individuals and families affected by asthma, and to raise the standard of care and quality of asthma education delivered to those with asthma. Links to top web resources for asthma are included on this web site.

Asthma and Allergy Foundation of America (AAFA)
1233 20th Street NW, Suite 402
Washington, DC 20036
Phone: 202/466-7643 or 800/727-8462
Web site: www.aafa.org

Resource for pamphlets, books and other materials on asthma and allergies with special emphasis on material for children and teens; videos and educational interactive CD-ROM games for children available; resource list and prices available upon request; bimonthly newsletter with AAFA membership.

Asthma Action America
Phone: 800/377-9575
Web site: www.asthmaactionamerica.org

Asthma Action America is a national asthma education campaign supported by leading organizations committed to improving healthcare. The goal of Asthma Action America is to increase awareness of asthma and effective asthma management. Supporting organizations include the AAAAI, AANP, AAPA, AARC, ACAAI, and many more. Web site contains an "asthma"

17

test, along with information concerning understanding asthma, what happens in the lungs, how to recognize symptoms, triggers, asthma categories, and myths and realities.

Asthma Society of Canada
130 Bridgeland Avenue, Suite 425
Toronto, Ontario M6A 1Z4 Canada
Phone: 866/787-4050 (Toll Free) or
          416/787-4050 (for Toronto residents)
Fax: 416/787-5807
Website: www.asthma.ca/adults

> Contains information for both children and adults regarding asthma, treatment, taking control, lifestyle, and resources and support information. Links to asthma education centers across Canada for people with asthma and their families to learn more about asthma.

Centers for Disease Control and Prevention (CDC)
1600 Clifton Road
Atlanta, GA 30333
Phone: 404/639-3311
Public Inquiries: 404/639-3534 or 800/311-3435
Web site: www.cdc.gov/asthma

> The CDC web site contains general information concerning asthma, including data and surveillance information. There is also a listing of links to web sites both within and outside of the CDC, together with information about air pollution and respiratory health.

European Respiratory Society (ERS)
4, Ave Sainte-Luce
CH-1003, Lausanne
Switzerland
Phone: +41 21 213 01 01
Web site: www.ersnet.org

> The ERS is the largest society in Europe in the field of respiratory medicine. Web site includes publications, educational, research, and meeting information for health care professionals.

Global Initiative for Asthma (GINA)
Web site: www.ginasthma.com

> GINA is a joint collaborative project between the National Heart, Lung and Blood Institute at the National Institutes of Health and the World Health Organization. GINA was created to help health-care professionals, public health officials and patients around the world reduce asthma prevalence, morbidity and mortality. It

prepares scientific reports on asthma management and prevention, encourages dissemination and adoption of the reports, and promotes international collaboration on asthma research.

The Lung Association
3 Raymond Street, Suite 300
Ottawa, ON K1R 1A3 Canada
Phone: 613/569-6411 or 888/566-LUNG (5864)
Fax: 613/569-8860
Web site: www.lung.ca
Asthma Resource Centre has information on asthma, allergies, management, asthma and exercise, asthma at school, asthma and pregnancy, nutrition, and medications.

**National Asthma Education and
Prevention Program (NAEPP)**
NHLBI Health Information Network
Attention: Web Site
PO Box 30105
Bethesda, MD 20824-0105
Phone: 301/592-8573 or 800/877-8339
Fax: 301/592-8563
Website: www.nhlbi.nih.gov
The NAEPP was initiated in March 1989 to address the growing problem of asthma in the United States. The NAEPP is administered and coordinated by the National Heart, Lung and Blood Institute. The NAEPP works with intermediaries, including major medical associations, voluntary health organizations, and community programs to educate patients, health professionals and the public. The ultimate goal of the NAEPP is to enhance the quality of life for patients with asthma and decrease asthma-related morbidity and mortality.The NAEPP distributes the Executive Summary of the NHLBI *Guidelines for the Diagnosis and Management of Asthma* free to the public, and provides information for patients, health professionals, schools, and the public.

National Heart, Lung, and Blood Institute
National Institutes of Health
PO Box 30105
Bethesda, MD 20824-0105
Phone: 301/592-8573
Fax: 301/592-8563
Web site: www.nhlbi.nih.gov
Information and booklets on controlling asthma and self-management of asthma; special publications and materials on

17

263

asthma for school administrators and school health workers. Also information for patients, general public, and health-care professionals.

National Institute of Allergy and Infectious Diseases
NIAID Office of Communications and Public Liaison
6610 Rockledge Drive, MSC 6612
Bethesda, MD 20892-6612
Phone: 301-496-5717
Fax: 301/402-3573
Web site: www3.niaid.nih.gov
   A division of the National Institutes of Health, this web site has information and statistics regarding asthma and allergy. Fact sheets and brochures on asthma and allergy are available as well as news releases and research information.

National Jewish Medical and Research Center
Global Leader in Lung, Allergic and Immune Diseases
1400 Jackson Street
Denver, CO 80206
Phone: 303/388-4461 or 800/222-LUNG (5864)
Web site: www.njc.org
   Toll-free number can be used to talk to a nurse about problems with asthma or for automated information; over a dozen booklets on understanding asthma and allergy available.

No Attacks (EPA-Ad Council)
Phone: 1-866-No-Attacks
Web site: www.noattacks.org
   Sponsored by the EPA and Ad Council, this web site contains information about asthma, in both English and Spanish. An asthma action plan is given, together with information on preventing attacks, an asthma hotline number, and a special section for kids.

Pulmonary Channel
136 West Street
Northampton, MA 01060
Phone: 888/950-0808 or 413/587-0244
Fax: 413/587-0387
Web site: www.pulmonologychannel.com/asthma
   This web site is physician developed and monitored, with information about asthma, self-management, frequently asked questions, and other aids.

Resource List for Asthma Education in the Schools

Available from the National Asthma Education Program, NHLBI Information Center, PO Box 30105 Bethesda, MD 20824-0105 (301/951-3260). This publication describes materials for educating teachers, health personnel and other school staff about asthma. Also for teaching children with asthma about asthma, how to manage it, and how to cope with it, and for educating families about asthma and how to help their children lead more normal lives.

World Health Organization (WHO)

Avenue Appia 20
1211 Geneva 27 Switzerland
Phone: +41 22 791 21 11
Fax: +41 22 791 3111
Web site: www.who.int/topics/asthma/en

The WHO web site contains links to descriptions of activities, reports, news, and events, as well as contacts and cooperating partners in the various WHO programs and offices working on asthma. Fact sheets are available online.

17

INDEX

Entries followed by *f* indicate figures; *t* indicates tables.

18

268

18

18

18

18

18

18

18

281

18

18

18